Essential Dental
Therapeutics

Essential Dental Therapeutics

Edited by

David Wray
University of Glasgow
UK

WILEY Blackwell

Registered Office(s): John Wiley & Sons, Inc., 111 River Street, Hoboken, NJ 07030, USA
John Wiley & Sons Ltd, The Atrium, Southern Gate, Chichester, West Sussex, PO19 8SQ, UK

Editorial Office: 9600 Garsington Road, Oxford, OX4 2DQ, UK

For details of our global editorial offices, customer services, and more information about Wiley products visit us at www.wiley.com.

Wiley also publishes its books in a variety of electronic formats and by print-on-demand. Some content that appears in standard print versions of this book may not be available in other formats.

Library of Congress Cataloging-in-Publication Data

Names: Wray, David, author.
Title: Essential dental therapeutics / by David Wray.
Description: First edition. | Chichester, West Sussex ; Hoboken : Wiley,
   2018. | Series: Essentials | Includes index. |
Identifiers: LCCN 2017014504 (print) | LCCN 2017015962 (ebook) | ISBN
   9781119057413 (pdf) | ISBN 9781119057420 (epub) | ISBN 9781119057390 (pbk.)
Subjects: | MESH: Dental Care | Drug Therapy
Classification: LCC RK51.5 (ebook) | LCC RK51.5 (print) | NLM WU 29 | DDC
   617.6–dc23
LC record available at https://lccn.loc.gov/2017014504

Cover design: Wiley
Cover image: © Vstock LLC/ Gettyimages

Set in 10/12pt, AGaramondPro by SPi Global, Chennai, India.
Printed and bound in Singapore by Markono Print Media Pte Ltd

10 9 8 7 6 5 4 3 2 1

Contents

List of contributors

Dr. Esther A. Hullah, BDS, MB ChB, MFDS RCS Eng, FDS (OM) RCS Eng, FHEA., Consultant and Specialist in Oral Medicine, Department of Oral Medicine, Guy's and St Thomas' NHS Foundation Trust & Honorary Lecturer in Oral Medicine, Kings College London Dental Institute, Guy's Hospital, London, United Kingdom

Dr Sabine Jurge, DDS, MSc, MBBS, MFDS RCS Eng, FDS (OM) RCPS, FHEA., Consultant and Specialist in Oral Medicine, Charles Clifford Dental Hospital, Sheffield Teaching Hospitals NHS Foundation Trust & Honorary Senior Clinical Lecturer in Oral Medicine, The School of Clinical Dentistry University of Sheffield, London, United Kingdom

Dr. Roddy McMillan, BDS, MB ChB, MFDS RCS Eng, FDS (OM) RCPS, FHEA., Consultant & Specialist in Oral Medicine, Eastman Dental Hospital, University College London Hospitals NHS Trust & Honorary Clinical Teaching Fellow in Oral Medicine and Facial Pain, Eastman Dental Institute, University College London, London, United Kingdom

Professor Alan J. Nimmo, PhD, BSc(Hons)., Professor of Medical Science, College of Medicine and Dentistry, James Cook University, Smithfield Campus, Cairns, Australia

Dr. Martyn Ormond, BDS, MBBS, MFDS RCS Ed., Specialty Registrar in Oral Medicine, Department of Oral Medicine, Guy's and St Thomas' NHS Foundation Trust & Honorary Lecturer in Oral Medicine, Department of Oral Medicine, Kings College London Dental Institute, Guy's Hospital, London, United Kingdom

Dr. Martina K. Shephard, BDent(Hons), MBBS(Hons), FRACDS, FDS (OM) RCS Eng., Consultant & Specialist in Oral Medicine, Eastman Dental Hospital, University College London Hospitals NHS Trust, London, United Kingdom

Dr. John C. Steele, BDS, MB ChB, MFDS RCS Ed, FDS (OM) RCS Ed, Dip OM, PGCTLCP, FHEA., Consultant & Specialist in Oral Medicine, The Leeds Teaching Hospitals NHS Trust & Honorary Senior Lecturer in Oral Medicine, Leeds Dental Institute, Faculty of Medicine & Health, University of Leeds, London, United Kingdom

Dr Jennifer Taylor, BDS, MB ChB, MFDS RCS Ed, FDS (OM) RCPS., Consultant and Specialist in Oral Medicine, Greater Glasgow and Clyde NHS Trust, &, Honorary Senior Lecturer in Oral Medicine, University of Glasgow, Glasgow Dental Hospital and School, 378 Sauchiehall Street, Glasgow, United Kingdom

Professor David Wray, MD(Hons), BDS, MB ChB, FDS RCPS, FDS RCS Ed, F Med Sci., Emeritus Professor, University of Glasgow, University Avenue, Glasgow, United Kingdom

Preface

Dentists, along with medical practitioners, are allowed to prescribe all medications although dentists must prescribe only within their competence as part of their clinical practice. Dentists, working within the National Health Service, are restricted to prescribing only those drugs included in the dental list and they must only prescribe generically.

Although the range of medications prescribed by dentists is narrower than their medical counterparts, dentists prescribe drugs to patients with a wide range of medical conditions who may be taking a number of other medications, which will influence dental practice as well as potentially causing interactions among the prescribed drugs.

For these reasons dentists must not only be familiar with the conditions they prescribe for and the drugs they prescribe but also they must be knowledgeable about general medical conditions affecting their patients and have knowledge of the drugs these patients may be concurrently taking.

To this end this textbook, designed to inform both dental students and dental practitioners, aims to provide information about dental prescribing and also general medical conditions, the drugs used to treat them, and their impact on dental practice.

This text does not cover the competencies required by the prescriber since these are detailed in the recently published Prescribing Competency Framework, produced the Royal Pharmaceutical Society under the aegis of NICE. The competencies contained in this Framework should be accomplished by all practitioners seeking to prescribe safely.

Similarly, this text does not detail specific prescribing details. These are comprehensively included in the *British National Formulary* and the *British National Formulary for Children* which are updated electronically, monthly and published in hard copy bi-annually and annually respectively. All prescribers should make reference to these sources when prescribing.

A specific, abridged text, *Drug Prescribing for Dentistry*, is produced by the Scottish Dental Clinical Effectiveness Programme (SDCEP.org.uk), which is also available as an iPhone app (https://itunes.apple.com/gb/app/sdcep-dental-prescribing/id509188306?mt=8). This provides explicit prescribing information for all drugs on the dental list and is designed to help dentists in primary care practice.

About the companion website

This book is accompanied by a companion website:

www.wiley.com/go/wray/dental-therapeutics

This website contains a set of multiple-choice questions for every chapter for students' use.

CHAPTER 1

Introduction to pharmacology and therapeutics – pharmacodynamics

Alan Nimmo

Key Topics

- Introduction to therapeutics – pharmacodynamics and the basis for drug action
- Molecular targets for drug action – receptors, enzymes, ion channels and carrier proteins
- Selective toxicity – the basis of antibacterial, antiviral and antifungal drug action, and cancer chemotherapy

Learning Objectives

- Be familiar with the main types of functional protein that serve as the molecular targets for drug action
- Be aware that in most cases, altering the activity of these proteins alters chemical signaling in the body, and hence control of body function
- Be familiar with how drugs, such as antibiotics, are able to exert a selectively toxic effect
- Be aware of the challenges posed in developing antiviral drugs and drugs for the treatment of cancer

Essential Dental Therapeutics, First Edition. Edited by David Wray.
© 2018 John Wiley & Sons Ltd. Published 2018 by John Wiley & Sons Ltd.
Companion Website: www.wiley.com/go/wray/dental-therapeutics

Introduction

Therapeutics has its roots in the historical use of herbal remedies and natural potions. However, the modern practice of therapeutics really began in the twentieth century. The herald for this new era was the German physician, Paul Ehrlich. Ehrlich sowed the seeds for transforming therapeutics into a science by insisting that drug action could be explained in terms of chemical and physical reactions. The understanding of how drugs produce their effects represents the area of therapeutics known as pharmacodynamics.

During the twentieth century, the advent of many effective therapeutic agents began to deliver immeasurable benefits to society. Perhaps the biggest single advance in medicine was the development of antibiotic therapies, exemplified by the work of Florey, Chain and Fleming on penicillin. The introduction of these novel treatments transformed what had previously been fatal or life-devastating diseases into manageable conditions.

However, we cannot be complacent. There are still many areas of practice where our current therapies have limited efficacy, or are associated with unwanted, or side, effects. For example, many cancer therapies come with significant side effects. In dental practice you'll see some of the most severe side effects associated with cancer treatment, such as stomatitis. It will only be through making cancer treatments more specific in the way they target cancerous cells, that we will be able to overcome many of these issues. Another challenge we face is the ability of bacteria to develop resistance to antibiotic therapy. In developed countries, antibiotic-resistant bacteria are now responsible for more deaths than HIV/AIDS. If we do not respond appropriately to these issues, we could return to an era where bacterial infections are no longer treatable. Hence therapeutics is, and needs to be, a constantly evolving science.

In dentistry, therapeutics may not be such a major component of daily practice as compared to general medical practice. However, an understanding of therapeutics is one of the cornerstones of good clinical dental practice. Pain-free dentistry would not be possible without the use of local anaesthetics, while analgesics are used to manage peri- and post-operative pain. In dental practice, the primary approach to managing microbial infection is surgical, however antibiotics do provide an important adjunct therapy, particularly in the case of a spreading infection. Dental practitioners also rely on drugs to manage fungal and viral infections, and inflammation. Other common uses of drugs in the dental clinic are to manage patient anxiety and to provide sedation for patients. However, this is only one side of the coin. Being aware of patients' general medical conditions, and their associated medications, is central to providing safe and effective treatment. Patients' medications may impact directly upon their oral health, for example many common medications cause the problem of xerostomia. In addition, medications may impact upon how a dentist manages a patient within the dental clinic. A significant number of patients may be receiving anticoagulant therapy in order to reduce their risk of a thrombotic event, such as a heart attack. However, a direct consequence of this is these patients will have a tendency to increased bleeding with surgical procedures, and this must be controlled with effective, local measures. Hence, good dental practice relies on a good understanding of therapeutics.

History of therapeutics

The practice of therapeutics is as old as history, and was well documented in ancient Greek and Egyptian civilizations. Throughout history there have been two opposing approaches to therapeutics, a magico-religious approach and an empirico-rational approach. The magico-religious approach is based upon the belief that disease is a supernatural event, and therefore should be managed by such forces, while the empirico-rational approach assumes that disease is a natural process that is best managed by a scientific approach, and evolving treatments in response to careful observation and evaluation of patient outcomes. It is this latter approach that forms the basis of current evidence-based practice.

In itself, the empirico-rational approach is not new. The father of modern medicine was the Ancient Greek physician, Hippocrates (circa 460–370 BCE). Hippocrates is accredited with insisting that disease is a natural process, and should be managed in a judicious manner. Some of the most basic principles of clinical practice, such as the importance of hygiene, can be traced back to the Hippocratic Works. Hippocrates even suggested that sometimes, 'to do nothing was the best remedy', recognition of the capacity of the human body to fight disease and initiate repair. However, for most of the intervening period between Hippocrates and the twentieth century, the practice of therapeutics was not based upon a scientific rationale. Common practices have included treatments such as bleeding patients, not only through the use of leeches, but also by severing blood vessels. Needless to say, many of these treatments did more harm than good. In fairness, though, a key underlying issue was that the function of the human body, and the basis of disease, was so poorly understood that it impeded a more scientific approach to medicine. It was the Russian physician, Virchow, who indicated that a scientific approach to therapeutics would come through its combination with physiology, and with it an improved understanding of normal body function.

As mentioned earlier, the historical basis of therapeutics lay in the use of natural potions, normally of plant origin. Some of these natural agents were actually very potent and effective. Indeed, there are a number of agents in current, clinical use, which have been used, in crude form, for hundreds, and even thousands of years. Some notable examples include the analgesic, morphine, which comes from the opium poppy, and the muscarinic antagonist, atropine, which comes from the plant, deadly nightshade. Indeed, the first local anaesthetic was cocaine, which comes from the leaves of the cocoa plant. One might assume that the existence of such effective medicinal agents would facilitate a scientific approach to therapeutics but, if anything, they tended to work against it. The issue was that those agents that were effective, produced their effects in such a specific and potent manner, that it was believed their actions could not be explained in terms of physical or chemical reactions. Instead, it was assumed that they must be imbued with some kind of magical, or vital forces. It was Paul Ehrlich, at the beginning of the twentieth century, who insisted that drug action should be understood in terms of normal chemical and physical reactions. In particular, he suggested that drugs are able to

produce their specific and selective effects because they bind to specific targets within the body. It is an understanding of these targets, and how drugs interact with them, that underpins modern pharmacology.

Targets for drug actions

Although there are hundreds of different drugs in clinical use, the way in which these drugs are able to produce their effects within the body is limited to a few basic mechanisms. Ehrlich suggested that drugs bind to specific target molecules, and we now recognize that these molecules are primarily key functional proteins, particularly proteins associated with communication within the body. The normal function of the body is under the control of the nervous, endocrine and paracrine systems. These systems use chemical mediators, such as neurotransmitters and hormones, to affect their control. In the same way, many drugs produce their effect by modulating this natural chemical signalling through targeting the functional proteins associated with chemical communication. The other, major way in which drugs act is by being selectively toxic, in other words they are toxic to particular cells or organisms, but are relatively innocuous to healthy human cells.

Receptors

As indicated, the key communication and control systems in the body exert their effects through the release of chemical mediators, such as neurotransmitters and hormones. These mediators are able to produce their effects on their target cells because those cells have receptors, that are not only capable of detecting chemical messages, but are also able to transduce and amplifying that signal to bring about a meaningful response within that cell. In terms of the way in which natural mediators act on these receptors, there are two components to their action. First, they bind to the receptor in question, but coupled to that, they also stimulate that receptor, to bring about a response. The ability of a messenger to bind to a particular receptor is referred to as its affinity, while the ability of the messenger to actually stimulate a receptor, and bring about a response, is referred to as efficacy. An analogy that is commonly used to describe this mechanism is the 'lock and key' effect. A key must not only have the correct shape to fit into a particular lock (affinity), but it must also have the precise shape that enables it to turn in the lock, and open that particular lock.

In terms of drugs, a number of drugs produce their effects by acting upon receptors, and thereby altering chemical signalling, and with it, control function within the body. Some drugs will produce their effect by mimicking the actions of the natural chemical messengers, in other words they will bind to, and stimulate the specific receptor. Those drugs, which have both affinity and efficacy for a particular receptor, are referred to as agonists. An example of a drug which acts as an agonist is salbutamol, which is used for the management of asthma. Salbutamol is an agonist for the beta2-adrenergic receptor. It mimics the natural actions of adrenaline on the beta2-receptors of airway smooth muscle, relaxing the airways, and thereby relieving an asthmatic attack.

Another way in which drugs can alter chemical signalling at receptors, is to block that receptor. If a drug binds to a receptor, but does not stimulate it, it has in itself no direct action. However, by binding to, and occupying the binding site, it can prevent the natural messenger from producing its effects at that receptor, and hence the drug can prevent a particular, unwanted response. Such drugs, which possess affinity for a receptor, but no efficacy, are referred to as antagonists. Such drugs are often identified by the prefix "anti" or the suffix "blocker", for example antihistamines or beta-blockers. Antihistamines can be used to manage some allergic reactions, such as allergic rhinitis, or hay fever, through blocking the unwanted actions of histamine.

Enzymes

The second class of functional protein that drugs may act upon, is enzymes. Enzymes are obviously essential for catalysing metabolic reactions within the body. However, a number of enzymes are responsible for the synthesis of, and degradation of, chemical messengers. It is particularly this kind of enzyme that serves as a target for drug activity.

The eicosanoids are a family of chemical messengers that are derived from membrane phospholipids. The synthesis of these mediators begins with the liberation of arachidonic acid from membrane phospholipids by the enzyme phospholipase A_2. The arachidonic acid is then metabolized by another enzyme, cyclooxygenase, to give rise to the prostanoids (prostaglandins and thromboxanes). These lipid mediators regulate a number of physiological processes, but are also important inflammatory mediators. The most widely used anti-inflammatory drugs are the non-steroidal anti-inflammatory drugs (NSAIDs), like ibuprofen. They produce their anti-inflammatory effects by inhibiting the cyclooxygenase enzyme, thereby inhibiting the production of the prostanoids.

Drugs that inhibit enzyme activity can also be used to enhance chemical signalling. Currently, the main agents used to manage Alzheimer's disease are acetylcholinesterase inhibitors. These drugs reduce the breakdown of acetylcholine, thereby increasing its activity in the brain.

Ion channels

The function of nerve and muscle cells is related to the electrical excitability of their cell membranes. For example, the ability of a nerve cell to send signals along the nerve axon is dependent upon its ability to generate action potentials. Membrane excitability is related to the presence of ion channels in the cell membrane. Drugs are able to modify the electrical activity of target cells by altering ion channel activity.

Local anaesthetics, like lignocaine, are the most widely used drugs within the dental clinic. Local anaesthetics produce their effects by blocking voltage-gated sodium ion channels. The opening of voltage-gated ion channels is central to the ability of a nerve to generate action potentials and, consequently, the ability of a nerve to signal. By blocking the transmembrane pore of the sodium ion channel, local anaesthetics inhibit the inward sodium current required to generate action potentials. As such, nociceptive nerves cannot send signals regarding a painful stimulus to the brain, and hence, pain sensations are abolished.

Drugs can also produce their effect by enhancing the opening of ion channels. For example, benzodiazepines, such as diazepam, which may be used as sedatives within the dental clinic, produce their effect by facilitating the opening of chloride ion channels associated with the $GABA_A$ receptor. GABA (γ-amino butyric acid) is the main inhibitory neurotransmitter in the brain, and its inhibitory effects are enhanced by benzodiazepines, which increase chloride ion channel opening, leading to hyperpolarization of neuronal cell membranes, and hence decreased excitability.

Carrier proteins

The fourth group of functional proteins that serve as a target for drugs are the carrier proteins associated with transmembrane transport. Again, for drugs that act on these targets, their main impact is on cell signalling and chemical communication.

In terms of nerve signalling, once a neurotransmitter has been released from a nerve terminal, there must be some mechanism to terminate the activity of the released neurotransmitter. This primarily happens in one of two ways. There may be enzymic breakdown of the released transmitter, as seen with acetylcholinesterase breaking down acetylcholine. Alternatively, a released neurotransmitter can be 'recycled' through neuronal reuptake involving a specific carrier protein. Such carrier proteins are responsible for the reuptake of catecholamines, such as noradrenaline and serotonin, following release. These carrier proteins serve as an important target for a number of anti-depressant medications. For example, drugs that inhibit the re-uptake of serotonin (selective serotonin reuptake inhibitors (SSRIs), e.g. fluoxetine), increase serotonin activity in the brain, and help enhance mood.

Selective toxicity

The other main way that drugs exert their beneficial effects is by being selectively toxic. As the name suggests, the drug should be toxic to a particular invading organism, but innocuous to healthy human cells. Selectively toxic agents form the basis for antibacterial, antiviral and antifungal drug treatments, as well as the treatment of cancer. The development of selectively toxic treatments relies on exploiting the biochemical differences between particular organisms

and cells. This may be 'relatively' easy when one is trying to deal with bacterial and fungal infections within a human, where there are significant differences between the organisms, but it becomes much more difficult when one tries to deal with viral infections and cancer.

Antibacterial drugs

There are significant biochemical differences between prokaryotic cells (bacteria) and mammalian, eukaryotic cells. A number of these serve as effective targets for antibacterial agents. Although not the first antibiotic, penicillin represented a major step forward in terms of being a very effective bactericidal agent. Penicillin, and all β-lactam antibiotics, such as amoxicillin, produce their effects by interfering with the synthesis and integrity of the bacterial cell wall. Because the main component of the bacterial cell wall, peptidoglycan, is not found in human cells, β-lactam antibiotics have a very low toxicity. However, some individuals may develop allergic reactions to penicillins. While severe allergic reactions and anaphylactic shock are rare, they may potentially be fatal.

There are other biochemical targets for antibiotic drugs. Some drugs, such as sulfonamides, can interfere with folic acid synthesis, which subsequently impacts upon nucleotide synthesis in bacterial cells, conferring a bacteriostatic effect. Other antibacterial agents, such as the tetracyclines, target protein synthesis, and in particular the differences between bacterial and mammalian ribosomes. The quinolones, such as ciprofloxacin, target a bacterial enzyme, known as topoisomerase II. These agents have become important in dealing with bacteria that are resistant to agents such as the penicillins.

Antifungal agents

There are a number of agents that can be used to manage fungal infections. Some of these agents, such as amphotericin and nystatin, are naturally occurring, while others, such as clotrimazole and fluconazole, are synthetic. Antifungal agents primarily target the fact that the fungal cell membrane contains the sterol, ergosterol, while animal cells, including humans, contains cholesterol.

Amphotericin and nystatin will preferentially bind to fungal cell membranes and form a transmembrane pore, disrupting the fungal cell. In contrast, the synthetic azoles still target ergosterol, but do so by inhibiting a fungal cytochrome enzyme responsible for ergosterol synthesis.

As a generalization, antifungal agents are safe and effective for use on topical, including oral infections, but require careful management when used for systemic infections in order to manage potential side effects.

Antiviral drugs

Historically, viral infections have been difficult to target with drug treatment. In themselves, viruses just consist of nucleic acid (either DNA or RNA) enclosed in a protein coat, or capsid. In order to replicate, viruses have to attach to, and enter a living, host cell. Having infected a host cell, the virus then uses the host cell's metabolic machinery to replicate. As such, there are very few biochemical differences between healthy human cells and those that are infected with a virus. However, in recent years, there has been a significant increase in the number of effective antiviral agents. This has occurred following the recognition that infected cells may contain virus-specific enzymes that are required for the replication and release of the virus particles. Aciclovir (zovirax) represented a major step forward in terms of developing effective antiviral agents. The drug itself is activated by one viral enzyme, viral thymidine kinase, and it subsequently inhibits another viral enzyme, viral DNA polymerase, that is required for viral replication. This two-step process gives aciclovir a high degree of selectivity in terms of inhibiting viral as opposed to human DNA polymerase. It is effective against infections caused by the herpes simplex and zoster viruses, including cold sores.

Cancer chemotherapy and treatment

Perhaps the hardest cells to target through a selectively toxic action are cancerous cells, since the biochemical differences between healthy and cancerous human cells are minimal. Historically, cancer treatments have primarily exerted a cytotoxic effect, targeting cells that are actively dividing. However, this does not represent a target that is selective for cancer, since many cells in the body are actively dividing in order to replace cells that have a high turnover rate. It is this, non-selective action that accounts for the many, significant side effects seen with cancer chemotherapy. Indeed, the epithelial cells that line the oral cavity have one of the highest turnover rates in the body, and as such, cancer chemotherapy can have marked effects in the oral cavity, causing problems such as stomatitis.

There is a constant drive to develop more selective drug treatments for cancer. Some success has been achieved by targeting growth-promoting signals that are overactive in some cancers. For example, in approximately 25% of breast cancers, the human epidermal growth factor receptor 2 is overexpressed, giving an increased growth-promoting stimulus (HER2+ve breast cancer). Trastuzumab (Herceptin) is a monoclonal antibody that binds to the HER2 receptor, and interferes with the growth stimulus produced by epidermal growth factor. However, perhaps the biggest conceptual breakthrough has come with the development of imatinib (Gleevec). Imatinib is a tyrosine-kinase inhibitor that is used in the treatment of a number of cancers, including chronic myelogenous leukemia. Imatinib inhibits a specific form of tyrosine kinase, BCR-Abl, which activates the signalling pathway responsible for the cancerous cells' growth. Because this tyrosine kinase is only found in certain cancerous cells, imatinib has a truly selectively toxic action against cancerous cells. As a result, imatinib is devoid of the significant side effects commonly associated with cancer treatment.

Conclusion

Antibiotic drugs, like penicillin helped revolutionize clinical practice, enabling the safe and effective management of conditions that had been previously fatal. Now, new antiviral and anticancer agents are showing that it is possible to achieve a similar, effective medical management of these conditions. However, we cannot be complacent, and we need strategies to manage problems like increasing antibiotic resistance in order to maintain the effectiveness of therapeutics.

CHAPTER 2

Introduction to pharmacology and therapeutics – pharmacokinetics

Alan Nimmo

Key Topics

- Introduction to pharmacokinetics and the factors that affect drug concentration within the body
- Drug diffusion and partitioning within the body
- Elimination of drugs from the body – metabolism and excretion
- Routes of drug administration
- Quantifying drug kinetics

Learning Objectives

- Be familiar with the factors that influence the concentration of a drug within the body
- Be aware of factors, such as regional differences in pH, which may influence the distribution of drugs within the body
- Be aware of the mechanisms involved in eliminating drugs from the body, and the potential for drug interactions and toxicity
- Be familiar with the main routes of drug administration
- Be aware of some of the basic approaches used to quantify drug kinetics

Essential Dental Therapeutics, First Edition. Edited by David Wray.
© 2018 John Wiley & Sons Ltd. Published 2018 by John Wiley & Sons Ltd.
Companion Website: www.wiley.com/go/wray/dental-therapeutics

Introduction

While the science of pharmacodynamics helps explain how drugs produce their effects within the body, safe clinical practice is equally dependent upon a knowledge of pharmacokinetics. By definition, pharmacokinetics studies the movement of drugs, and in particular their ability to move from their site of administration to their site of action. However, it is also the science that determines the correct dose and route of administration of a particular drug in order to ensure that one achieves the required concentration of the drug at its target site.

The importance of correct dosing cannot be overstated. Drugs will only produce their beneficial effects within their 'therapeutic range'. If the drug concentration is too low, then the required, beneficial effects will not be achieved, while if the dose is too high, unwanted or toxic effects of the drug will start to predominate. For some drugs, their therapeutic range may be quite wide, making them both easy and safe to use in clinical practice. However, other drugs may have a narrow therapeutic range, requiring careful management and monitoring in order to avoid adverse reactions. In the words of the Swiss-German physician Paracelsus (1493–1541), who has been credited as the founder of modern toxicology, 'Solely the dose determines that a thing is not a poison'.

There is a whole range of factors that will influence the concentration of a drug at its target site and, in general, they are all interdependent. These factors are commonly divided into four components, referred to as the phases of drug disposition, these being absorption, distribution, metabolism and excretion, commonly abbreviated to ADME. When one thinks about administering a local anaesthetic in the dental clinic, one may feel that these factors are of little importance, since the drug is being 'placed' near the nerve you want to block. However, you will find it is much more difficult to achieve effective anaesthesia in an area where there is significant inflammation, as compared to non-inflamed tissue. One potential explanation for this lies in an understanding of basic pharmacokinetics.

Introduction to pharmacokinetics

While absorption is considered the first phase of drug disposition, it is perhaps worth considering the factors that affect drug distribution first of all, since these can have broad ramifications, including influencing the route of administration.

Distribution

For many drugs, following administration, they are transported around the body via the bloodstream. Drugs may be either injected directly into the circulation (i.e. intravenous injection), or they may enter the circulation, for example following absorption from the gastrointestinal tract. Once in the bloodstream, almost all drugs are transported in exactly the same way, by what is referred to as bulk-flow transfer, where the drug is transported rapidly around the body. Because most drugs are transported in the same way, this does not have a major influence on the pharmacokinetic characteristics of an individual drug. The one caveat to that is that within the bloodstream, many drugs will bind to the plasma proteins, which will influence their movement, but we will discuss this aspect separately. However, for a drug to produce its effects within the body, it will have to leave the bloodstream and diffuse to its target site. It is this ability of a drug to diffuse within the body that is a key factor in determining an individual drug's pharmacokinetic properties.

In order to understand the way a drug is able to move around the body, perhaps the first thing that needs to be considered is the nature of the body itself. Our body does not consist of one single compartment, but instead is made up of a number of different compartments, each with its own physicochemical characteristics. The barriers that separate these various compartments are composed of our body's cells, for example epithelial cells lining the gastrointestinal tract. With these cellular barriers, it is the phospholipid membrane of the cell that forms the actual barrier. For a drug to pass through such a barrier, there are two possibilities.

On the one hand, a drug may pass between the cells if there are gaps between neighbouring cells forming the barrier (paracellular movement). This is seen in many capillaries, where there are small pores, or intercellular clefts, between the vascular endothelial cells. These pores allow for the passage of small, water-soluble molecules through the barrier. However, larger molecules, such as plasma proteins, are too big to pass through these pores, and will be retained in the circulation.

However, other barriers, such as the blood-brain barrier, serve a protective function, and here there are tight junctions between neighbouring cells, giving the barrier more functional integrity. For a drug to cross such a barrier, it has to be able to pass through the cells (transcellular movement), rather than between them. The blood-brain barrier represents the most robust barrier within the body, with astrocyte foot processes providing an extra cell layer around the vascular endothelium to both restrict and regulate the movement of solutes.

There are four basic ways in which a drug molecule may diffuse through an epithelial or endothelial cell barrier. If the drug molecule is neither ionized nor polar, then the molecule will have sufficient lipid solubility to diffuse directly through the cell membrane. However, many drugs are either weak acids or bases, and hence, at any one time, exist in both an ionized and non-ionized form. The actual proportion of these forms, and therefore the overall lipid solubility of the drug, will depend upon the pH of the solution in which the drug is dissolved. We will revisit this concept in considering pH partitioning.

The second mechanism by which drugs can cross a cell membrane is in combination with a carrier protein that either facilitates diffusion, or enables active transport. Such carriers naturally transport endogenous chemicals, such as nutrients, but may also facilitate drug movement. These carriers are mainly confined to specific organs, such as the gastrointestinal tract and kidney, and are also important in blood-brain barrier function.

Thirdly, drugs can transverse the cell membrane by the process of pinocytosis, or 'cell drinking', where the cell membrane invaginates around the molecule forming a vesicle, which is then transported into the cell. Pinocytosis may assist larger molecules, such as insulin, to cross the blood-brain barrier, but is unlikely to assist the transport of small drug molecules.

Finally, the presence of aqueous pores (aquaporins) and ion channels may potentially enable the movement of very small molecules or ions, such as lithium, to enter the intracellular fluid. However, in general, lipid diffusion and carrier-mediated transport are the more important mechanisms for the transcellular movement of drugs.

Partitioning:

As mentioned, the body not only contains a variety of compartments, but those compartments have different physicochemical properties. For example, the plasma of the bloodstream is a protein-rich aqueous solution, while adipose tissue represents a predominantly lipid environment. The pH of the plasma in the bloodstream is very slightly alkaline (pH 7.4), while gastric acid makes the lumen of the stomach highly acidic (~pH 2). These different chemical environments can lead to an uneven distribution of a drug within the body because, depending upon the chemical nature of a drug, it may have a greater affinity for one environment over another. The main factors that give rise to an uneven drug distribution within the body are pH differences across a barrier (pH partitioning), protein binding and sequestration into lipid.

pH Partitioning:

For most drugs to diffuse through the barriers between compartments within the body, they must be in a non-ionized, and hence lipid soluble form. However, because many drugs are weak acids or bases, they exist in both an ionized and non-ionized state. The proportion of the two forms will vary depending upon the pH of the solution in which it is dissolved. For example, if a weak acid is dissolved in an acidic solution, it will be predominantly non-ionized, as compared to when it is in a basic solution, where it will be mostly ionized. The converse is the case for a weak base, which will be predominantly ionized in an acidic solution. If one knows the dissociation constant, or pKa, of the drug in question, the precise proportion of the two forms can be calculated using the Henderson-Hasselbach equation. It is worth keeping in mind that the pKa does not indicate whether a drug is a weak acid or base, but rather indicates its tendency to dissociate, depending upon the pH of its environment.

pH partitioning occurs when one has solutions of different pH on either side of a barrier. Within the human body, this occurs most markedly between the lumen of the stomach and the bloodstream. Keeping in mind that only the non-ionized form of the drug can diffuse through the barrier, the concentration gradients that drive diffusion only relate to the non-ionized form. Hence, if you have a weak acid in an acidic environment, the concentration of the non-ionized form is high, while in an alkaline environment, the non-ionized form has a low concentration. This provides a driving force for diffusion. As a result, weak acids tend to move from a relatively acidic environment to a more alkaline one. The opposite happens with weak bases, where they tend to diffuse from a more alkaline environment to an acidic one.

From a dentistry perspective, pH partitioning may impact upon local anaesthesia when there is significant, local inflammation. By nature, local anaesthetics are weak bases. It is the ionized form of the anaesthetic that interacts with the binding site in the transmembrane pore of the voltage-gated Na^+ ion channel to produce the blockade. Access to the channel's binding site can occur either by direct diffusion through the neuronal membrane (hydrophobic pathway) or by first diffusing through the membrane into the cytoplasm, and then entering the active channel from the intracellular compartment (hydrophilic pathway). Both of these pathways rely on having a sufficient concentration of the non-ionized form of the anaesthetic outside the nerve, to drive diffusion through the neuronal membrane. Unfortunately, inflammation may cause the extracellular fluid to become more acid, reducing the concentration of the non-ionized form of the anaesthetic, thereby reducing diffusion of the anaesthetic into the nerve.

Protein binding:

In addition to acting on their target proteins, drugs may bind to other proteins, most notably the plasma protein, albumin. As a generalization, acidic drugs, such as NSAIDs, tend to bind more readily to plasma albumin than basic drugs, but there are a number of basic drugs, such as tricyclic antidepressants, that do bind. For some drugs, a significant proportion of the drug within the bloodstream may be bound to the plasma proteins (e.g. 99%), while only a small proportion is in free solution. This has a number of implications. Since the pores in the vascular endothelium are relatively small, plasma proteins, and with them the bound fraction of the drug, remain in the bloodstream, while only the drug in free solution is able to diffuse out of the circulation in order to produce its effects. For drugs with a high degree of protein binding, a significant proportion of the total drug within the body is retained in the circulation. In this way, plasma proteins can act as a 'slow release' mechanism for certain medications. The portion of a drug that is bound to the plasma proteins is also 'protected' from metabolism and excretion.

The other key aspect in relation to protein binding is it provides one mechanism by which drug–drug interactions can occur. Each albumin molecule has two drug-binding sites, and the concentration of albumin in the plasma is approximately 0.6 mmol/l. Given that most drugs produce their effects at relatively low concentrations (e.g. $1\mu M$), there is an abundance of binding sites. However, for drugs that act at relatively high concentrations and exhibit a high degree of protein binding, there is the potential for competition for binding sites, and for one drug to displace another from plasma proteins. For drugs that are normally highly bound to plasma proteins, even the displacement of a relatively small proportion of the bound drug can have a huge impact on the concentration of the free drug, and with that, greatly increase the effects of the drug.

Sequestration into lipid:

Approximately 20% of our body mass is lipid. As indicated, many drugs need to be reasonably lipid soluble in order to reach their target sites within the body, and this is particularly true of drugs that are able to act on the CNS. As such, these drugs must have some tendency to enter the lipid compartments in the body. However, for most of these drugs, they are not so lipid soluble that there is any significant sequestration into body fat. The main exception to this is general anaesthetics, which rely on high lipid solubility for their anaesthetic potency. General anaesthetics will tend to accumulate in body fat, and this is responsible for both the slow onset of action, and slow recovery, that is seen with inhaled anaesthetics.

Elimination of drugs from the body

Most drugs are eliminated from the body by renal excretion. However, the kidneys are much more efficient at excreting water-soluble wastes as compared to lipid-soluble ones. As such, the body's ability to excrete more lipophilic agents occurs in two stages. First, these drugs will undergo metabolic alteration in order to generate metabolites that are more water-soluble than the parent drug. These water-soluble metabolites can then be excreted by the kidneys.

Metabolism:

Drug metabolism predominantly occurs within the liver, although there are enzymes in other tissues, including the plasma, that have a metabolic potential. Depending upon the local anaesthetic used, both aspects of metabolism are important. Local anaesthetics that contain an ester bond, such as benzocaine, are rapidly metabolized by plasma esterases, while those containing an amide bond, such as lignocaine, are metabolized by hepatic amidases, giving them a longer half-life.

Drug metabolism primarily occurs as a two-step process, involving two types of metabolic reaction, referred to as Phase I and Phase II reactions. These two reactions occur in a sequential manner. Phase I reactions involve processes such as oxidation and reduction, which make the drug more chemically reactive, and sometimes more toxic. These are followed by a second set of reactions (Phase II), which involve conjugation. The addition of a chemical substituent on to the molecule renders the drug more water soluble, as well as normally abolishing activity.

While metabolism normally provides a mechanism for abolishing drug activity, there are a few drugs that are administered in an inactive form, and rely on metabolism to convert them into the active form, for example the corticosteroid, prednisone needs to be converted into its active form, prednisolone.

The other potential issue around drug metabolism is toxicity. Toxic metabolites may be generated by the Phase I reactions, but while they are rapidly 'mopped-up' by the Phase II reactions, they do not normally pose an issue. However, in certain situations, such as drug overdose, the toxic, Phase I metabolites may be generated more rapidly than they are removed, giving the potential to cause harm. Perhaps, not surprisingly, the liver is one of the main victims in this situation, since these toxic metabolites are at their highest concentration in the liver. This situation is epitomized with paracetamol, where the parent drug is a very safe agent. However, in an overdose situation, the hydroxylated metabolite builds up, potentially causing liver damage or failure.

Excretion:

Renal excretion is the main route of elimination of drugs from the body. However, there are significant differences in the way the kidneys handle different drugs.

Drugs in free solution (i.e. not bound to plasma proteins) are readily filtered in the kidneys, and enter the glomerular filtrate in the nephron. As the filtrate passes through the nephron its composition, including drug concentration, are markedly altered by the processes of tubular reabsorption and secretion. Some drugs, particularly those that are relatively lipid soluble, may diffuse from the renal tubule back into the circulation, resulting in slow renal excretion. In contrast, some drugs are actively secreted from the circulation into the forming urine in the renal tubules, resulting in rapid renal excretion. The antibiotic, penicillin, is particularly susceptible to this rapid renal clearance as a result of tubular secretion. However, this rapid elimination of penicillin can be prevented by formulating it with a drug, such as probenecid, that competes for the renal transport protein.

In addition to renal excretion, drugs may also be removed from the body by excretion into bile, and subsequent elimination in faeces, as well as by exhalation. Exhalation is the main route of elimination of gaseous, or volatile, anaesthetics, as well as the inhaled dental sedative, nitrous oxide.

Routes of administration and drug absorption

There are a number of different routes of administration available for medications, each with their own benefits and limitations. In general, the most popular route for drug administration is the oral route. However, the popularity of oral administration reflects patient preference and compliance, rather than the effectiveness of the route. Indeed, there are a whole range of factors that impact upon the absorption of drugs from the gastrointestinal (GI) tract.

Agents taken orally are subject to the acidic environment of the stomach, as well as the digestive enzymes found in the GI tract. The rate of transit of a drug through the gut, and hence rate of absorption, is affected by GI motility, which may be influenced by food intake, disease and other medications. Absorption from the gut is also influenced by splanchnic blood flow, as well as the potential for interactions with GI contents. For example, the absorption of tetracycline antibiotics can be inhibited by Ca^{2+} ions. However, perhaps the most significant issue with oral administration, is that substances absorbed from the GI tract enter the hepatic circulation, and travel to the liver prior to entering the systemic circulation. As mentioned, the liver is the main site of drug metabolism and, as a result, significant amounts of a drug may be metabolized before reaching the systemic circulation, giving rise to a phenomenon known as first-pass, or pre-systemic metabolism. While one can compensate for this metabolism by administering increased amounts of a drug, this leads to increased levels of metabolites, and potential unwanted effects.

Injection represents a more reliable route of administration. For systemic drug action, intravenous injection provides certainty over how much drug entered the systemic circulation and when. Other effective, but slower routes of systemic administration, are intramuscular and subcutaneous injections, where the drug is absorbed from the site of injection, into the circulation. The rate of absorption will depend upon factors such as local blood flow. Injections also provide a mechanism for topical, or local, effects, as with local anaesthesia in dentistry. The local actions of the anaesthetic may be enhanced by formulating it with a vasoconstrictor, such as adrenaline, in order to reduce local blood flow, and retain the anaesthetic at the site of administration.

Volatile agents, such as gaseous general anaesthetics and nitrous oxide, can be administered by inhalation. These gases can quickly equilibrate between alveolar air and arterial blood particularly if, like nitrous oxide, they have a low solubility. Drugs may also be absorbed through mucous membranes, enabling topical effects of agents within the oral cavity. However, sublingual and buccal administration may also be used for systemic administration, with the advantage that the drug is absorbed directly into the systemic circulation, by-passing pre-systemic metabolism. A similar effect may be achieved through rectal administration.

Basic kinetics

While the ability of a drug to get to its target site and start producing its beneficial effects is a key consideration, we do also have to consider how a drug is eliminated from the body. The dosing, and dosing regimen of a drug is determined by both the absorption of a drug by the body, and its subsequent elimination. A detailed consideration of drug kinetics is beyond the scope of this chapter, but we will introduce some key terms and concepts.

The rate at which a drug is eliminated from the body is normally expressed as the rate of clearance (CL). As mentioned, drugs may be cleared from the body by different routes, such as renal excretion or metabolism. The overall clearance of a drug (CL_{tot}) represents the sum of the different routes of clearance, for example $CL_{ren} + CL_{met}$ would account for elimination by both renal excretion and metabolism. The way in which clearance is expressed (ml/min or l/h) is best understood by thinking about renal clearance (CL_{ren}). The rate at which a drug is being eliminated by the kidneys is related to its concentration in the urine (C_u), and the volume of urine (V_u) that is produced in a particular time. This rate of elimination also needs to be related to the amount of drug in the body, reflected by its plasma concentration (C_p). The units of clearance, such as ml/min, reflect the volume of plasma that would be cleared of the drug in that particular time.

$$CL_{ren} = (C_u \times V_u) / C_p \qquad (2.1)$$

The same concepts and units apply to overall drug clearance (CL_{tot}) by the body, in other words, the volume of plasma that would be cleared of a drug in a given time.

In terms of quantifying drug kinetics in order to inform drug dosing, a common approach is to talk about a drug's half-life, or half-rate of elimination. For many drugs, their rate of elimination exhibits 'first-order kinetics', which means that the rate of elimination is directly proportional to the drug concentration – the higher the drug concentration, the more rapidly it is eliminated from the body. Following the administration of a single dose of such a drug, its elimination from, and resultant concentration in the body follows an exponential decay. The elimination half-life is the time taken for the plasma concentration to fall by half. After a subsequent half-life, the concentration fall by another half (i.e. one-quarter of the original plasma concentration), and so on.

While there are situations where a single dose of a drug may be administered, often patients will receive a course of medication involving repeated doses. Repeated doses are normally given at intervals that are approximately equal to the drug's half-life. In such situations, the new dose superimposes upon the existing amount of the drug in the body, giving a new, higher concentration. However, after approximately four doses, a 'steady state' is achieved, where the rate at which the drug is being administered is equal to the rate at which it is being eliminated from the body.

Not all drugs follow this exponential fall in concentration. For some drugs, such as alcohol, where enzymatic degradation or carrier-mediated elimination are important, these mechanisms may have a limited, or finite, capacity to remove the drug, and therefore the elimination occurs at a steady rate. This is referred to as saturation, or zero-order, kinetics.

In terms of drug kinetics, the plasma concentration of a drug plays an important role in determining its kinetic characteristics. However, as mentioned earlier, many drugs are not evenly distributed within the body. One way of quantifying this partitioning is to talk about the volume of distribution of a drug. The volume of distribution (V_d) is basically the total amount of drug administered (Q), divided by its plasma concentration (C_p):

$$V_d = Q / C_p \qquad (2.2)$$

If most of the drug remains within the circulation (e.g. as a result of protein binding), the plasma concentration will be high, and hence the volume of distribution will be low. Conversely, if most of the drug leaves the circulation, the plasma concentration will be low, and hence the volume of distribution will be high. The volume of distribution provides a way of relating the amount of drug administered to its plasma concentration.

CHAPTER 3

Introduction to pharmacology and therapeutics – drug safety

Alan Nimmo

Key Topics

- Introduction to the factors that underlie safe drug prescribing
- Extension and side effects associated with drug therapy, and allergic reactions
- Drug safety issues during pregnancy
- Clinical studies to determine safety and effectiveness of drug therapies
- Individual reactions to drug treatment

Learning Objectives

- Be familiar with the basic factors that underpin safe prescribing
- Be familiar with the adverse reactions that may occur with drug therapies, and the distinction between extension and side effects
- Be aware of the increased need for vigilance in drug prescribing if a patient may be pregnant, and also in elderly patients where polypharmacy may be an issue
- Be aware of the need for pharmacovigilance
- Be aware of the potential for individual variations in response to drug treatment

Essential Dental Therapeutics, First Edition. Edited by David Wray.
© 2018 John Wiley & Sons Ltd. Published 2018 by John Wiley & Sons Ltd.
Companion Website: www.wiley.com/go/wray/dental-therapeutics

Introduction

By definition, a drug is a chemical that changes the function of the body. Obviously, the aim of drug therapy is to use these agents to achieve a positive, or beneficial outcome for the patient. The benefit derived may range from making the patient's visit to the dental clinic more comfortable, through to treating a potentially life-threatening infection. However, when used inappropriately, the effect a drug has on the body may be undesirable, and hence its effects are more akin to a poison. There is really nothing inherent about a drug that makes it either safe or unsafe, it comes down to the skill of the clinician combined with careful, informed prescribing that ensures the best clinical outcomes for their patients. The benefits delivered by a drug depend upon when it is used, why it is used, how it is used, how much is used, and whether there are other drugs being used at the same time. There are also individual patient factors that may come into play.

Regulatory authorities employ a rigorous registration process to help ensure that new medications demonstrate acceptable levels of both safety and efficacy. However, the onus is still on the clinician to use these drugs in a way that optimizes the beneficial effects. A clinician must use all the current, available evidence to make their prescribing choices. The complexity of these issues may be illustrated in relation to the use of antibiotics, such as penicillin. Antibiotics save millions of lives every year, and we tend now to take for granted the benefits they produce. However, a small percentage of the population are allergic to penicillins, and severe, penicillin-induced anaphylaxis accounts for more than one thousand deaths per year. While antibiotics are primarily used to treat a confirmed bacterial infection, a proportion of the patient population may benefit from prophylactic antibiotic therapy to avoid iatrogenic infection. Finally, the development of multi-drug resistant strains of bacteria is becoming a major concern, and this is partly fuelled by the over-use of antibiotics, and may be compounded in some cases by poor patient compliance. Hence, appropriate prescribing requires all of these benefits and risks to be balanced in light of current clinical evidence.

While drug prescribing is a smaller component of dental practice as opposed to medical practice, the dental practitioner must be aware of all the potential issues around, not just the medications they use and prescribe, but also any other medications their patients may be taking.

Determining drug safety

Therapeutic index

Safe and effective drug prescribing is basically informed by risk-benefit analyses. One commonly used measure of that balance is the therapeutic index, which is determined by the lethal dose in 50% of a population (LD_{50}) divided by the effective dose, again for 50% of a population (ED_{50}). Basically, the larger the therapeutic index, the safer the drug is, at least in theory. In other words, the bigger the difference between the dose required to produce the beneficial effects of the drug, as compared to its toxic effects, the greater the margin of safety. However, there are a number of significant limitations to this measure. First, the LD_{50} value is not a clinical measurement, but rather is derived from animal studies. In addition, a measure like LD_{50} does not necessarily reflect the kind of adverse effects that one may see in the clinic. For example, from its therapeutic index, penicillin is an extremely safe drug. Unfortunately, the risk of allergic reactions is not reflected by this measure. In a similar manner, perhaps the most notorious drug in the history of medicine, thalidomide, also has a very high therapeutic index. Its capacity to cause gross malformations in the developing foetus is not reflected by this 'safety' measure.

Extension and side effects with drug therapy

All drugs have the potential to produce harmful as well as beneficial effects, and most commonly, any unwanted effects are normally related to the main mechanism of action of the drug. As such, many of these adverse events are predictable once one understands the mechanism of action of the drug. Often the unwanted effects simply reflect the basic action of the drug. For example, a common issue with sedative drugs is tendency to cause drowsiness, or anti-coagulant therapies may cause excessive bleeding. Such problems are referred to as extension effects, and are commonly associated with higher doses of the drug. Such reactions are predictable, and in most cases the problems can be prevented by appropriate dosing, or may be reversed by reducing the dose.

Drugs may also produce adverse effects that are unrelated to the therapeutic goal of the treatment, and these are referred to as side effects. In many cases these effects may be both predictable and dose-dependent. One of the goals of drug development is to try to enhance the beneficial effects of a drug, while reducing the unwanted effects. The development of bronchodilators for the treatment of asthma illustrates how drug therapy can be improved by a better understanding of the molecular and cellular action of drugs. The first synthetic bronchodilator to be developed was isoprenaline, a non-selective beta-adrenergic agonist. Isoprenaline stimulates both $\beta 1$ and $\beta 2$ adrenergic receptors. Stimulation of the $\beta 2$-adrenoceptors on airway smooth muscle produces bronchodilation, and hence delivers the beneficial effects of the therapy. However, stimulation of the $\beta 1$-adrenoceptors on the heart will cause tachycardia and palpatations, which is unpleasant, and potentially dangerous in some patients. The cardiac effects are predictable, given the nature of the drug, but are also unwanted. The subsequent development of selective $\beta 2$ agonists, such as salbutamol, resulted in the beneficial effects of the bronchodilator being retained, while the cardiovascular side effects were significantly reduced. However, it is not always so straightforward to reduce unwanted effects. Opioid analgesics, such as morphine, have a tendency to cause nausea and vomiting in approximately 40% of patients. However, this tendency to cause nausea and vomiting appears to be inseparable from the analgesic effects, and occurs at the same doses.

Unfortunately, sometimes we have little choice but to tolerate side effects, because there are no viable alternatives available. For example, the side effects with cancer chemotherapy are often very severe but, in terms of a risk–benefit decision, our choices are limited. However, on-going research and development is starting to yield effective cancer treatments, such as imatinib, which exhibit a significantly improved beneficial–side effect profile.

From the dentistry perspective, probably one of the most common issues associated with systemic medication is the problem of xerostomia, and therefore one must examine ways of minimizing the impact this may have on one's patients.

Drug allergy

Approximately 10% of all untoward drug reactions have an allergic component. There are a number of characteristics that tend to distinguish allergic drug reactions from other untoward events. First, for an allergic response to occur, there must have been prior exposure to the same drug, or at least a closely related compound. Unlike side effects, the severity of the allergic reaction is seemingly independent of the dose of the drug. This occurs because the response is not produced by the drug itself, but rather the body's immune response to it. Some drugs never cause allergies while others have had to be withdrawn from the clinic because they are too allergenic. Some of the most common allergic reactions are associated with antibiotics. The incidence of allergic responses to drugs like penicillin and sulfonamides is around 5% in the general population.

Most allergic drug reactions are mild, such as development of a rash. Thankfully, serious reactions, such as anaphylaxis, are rare, but they can be fatal. Penicillin is the most common cause of drug-induced anaphylaxis, with an incidence rate of about 1 in 50,000 patients. As mentioned before, such allergic reactions are not related to the dose of the drug, and a patient has been known to die following a topical application of less than 1 µg of penicillin. As a dental practitioner, you must be able to manage such an immediate anaphylactic reaction without medical back-up. While drug allergy cannot always be prevented, the risks posed can be minimized by good clinical practices, such as ensuring you have an adequate medical history, and avoiding not just the offending drug, but also likely cross-reactors.

Drugs in pregnancy

As discussed in Chapter 14, standard dental treatment is not only safe, but is advisable, throughout pregnancy. However, extreme care must always be exercised in terms of drug prescribing during pregnancy, and certain drugs, such as benzodiazepines, must be avoided. That said, drugs are still widely used during pregnancy, since the health of the developing foetus does depend upon maternal health. While the first trimester of pregnancy is the most critical, drug-related issues can occur throughout pregnancy.

Some drugs, like benzodiazepine sedatives, can cause gross structural malformations during foetal development. Such agents are referred to as teratogens. Such drugs impact upon normal organogenesis, giving rise to developmental defects in one, or more, areas. If these defects are incompatible with life, this will lead to foetal death. However, if the defects are less severe, the child will be born with malformations. The specific malformations that occur will depend upon the action of the drug and the time in pregnancy at which it was administered. Gross malformations are more likely to occur when drugs are administered in early pregnancy, but normal development can be affected anytime during pregnancy. While the causes of oral clefts are multifactorial, the consumption of alcohol or some anti-epileptic medications, such as valproic acid, during the first trimester of pregnancy may increase the risk of clefting.

Natural therapies

In terms of taking an accurate medication history, it is vital that you not only get information regarding a patient's prescribed medication, but also any over-the-counter medications and natural remedies they may be taking. Unfortunately, many patients view natural therapies as being 'safe' alternatives, but these agents can play just as significant a role in terms of drug–drug interactions as any prescribed medication. For example, St John's wort, which has been clinically validated as an effective mild anti-depressant drug, can pose significant issues in medical practice in relation to drug–drug interactions. The issues may not be as significant in dental practice, but they still need to be noted. If a benzodiazepine is being used as a sedative, St John's wort will increase its hepatic metabolism and reduce its effectiveness. Conversely, garlic tablets, which are sometimes taken to relieve cold and flu symptoms, can reduce the metabolism of benzodiazepines, causing increased sedation.

Clinical studies

Improved healthcare is totally dependent upon on-going research and clinical studies. Such studies may look at optimizing existing treatments to improve patient outcomes, or be used to introduce new treatments into the clinic. The introduction of a new drug into the clinic is a very long and expensive process, where ethical and safety concerns are just as paramount as the effectiveness of the new treatment. It is estimated that it costs more than US$2.5 billion to bring a new prescription drug to the clinic. Before any new drug is tested on a patient, it undergoes many years of pre-clinical research to primarily establish its safety profile, but also examine its potential to bring positive therapeutic outcomes.

Clinical trials of a new drug are divided into four phases, Phase 1–4. For most new drugs, with cancer treatments being the obvious exception, Phase 1 involves testing the drug in healthy human volunteers to examine the safety and pharmacokinetic properties of the drug, including safe dose levels. Phase 2 is normally the first trial of the drug in the target patient population, where it may be trialed on up to a few hundred patients. These studies look at the safety of the drug in the patient population, as well as providing the first indications of the effectiveness of the drug. Phase 3 studies may look at around 1000 patients, and are aimed at establishing the effectiveness of the drug as compared to existing treatments, as well as its safety in a large cohort. Once a new drug is approved following Phase 3, its safety and effectiveness observed in a larger patient group (Phase 4), which may involve as many as 10,000 or more patients.

The value of a new treatment can only be assessed if it can be compared to a patient not receiving treatment, or receiving an existing treatment. Obviously, there are ethical issues around the former, unless no effective treatment currently exists. Hence, a trial should compare two groups, a control and a test group. In order to avoid the potential for biasing the results of a clinical study, a number of strategies may be used. First, patients should be randomly assigned to a particular group. Second, neither the patient nor the clinician should be aware of what treatment a particular patient is receiving until after the study is concluded (double-blind study). In a controlled trial, a placebo, or 'dummy' treatment may be used to ensure that the patient is unaware of whether they are receiving treatment or not. Sometimes patients may show a positive response to a placebo because they believe the treatment is beneficial to them, the so-called 'placebo-response'.

Meta analysis

Sometimes the results of individual clinical studies may appear to be contradictory, or give mixed messages. One way of trying to achieve an objective view from a number of individual studies is to perform a meta-analysis. Combining the results of multiple trials, and with that increasing the size of the patient sample, gives more statistical power as compared to smaller, individual trials. The value of the meta-analysis however depends upon the quality of design of the original studies. In addition, since the data used for meta-analysis comes from published results, it may be affected by 'publication bias', since, as a generalization, it is easier to publish positive results as compared to negative ones.

Pharmacovigilance

While drug safety is a paramount consideration with clinical trials, by their nature these trials involve a very small percentage of the total patient population. As such, the full safety profile of a drug is often not known until it has been used in the clinic for a number of years. Some adverse events may be very rare, only being seen in 1 in 10,000 patients. Additional safety data can be gathered from on-going, large-cohort studies. However, it is also important that any adverse drug reactions are reported in order to ensure that such events, however rare, are noted. The reporting of adverse events is particularly important for new medications, but it should still happen when more serious reactions to well-established medications are observed.

Individual variations

We recognize that all patients are individuals, and therefore it should not be surprising that their responses to medications will vary as well. Our genetic make-up will influence how we respond to a particular drug treatment. As such, there is an increasing interest in the field of pharmacogenetics, since this may help to identify which patients may benefit from a particular treatment, or which patients may be at risk of adverse reactions.

Most commonly, genetic influences on drug responses follow a continuous, or 'normal', distribution pattern, similar to other population characteristics like height or weight. However, occasionally one may get discontinuous variation. For example, unlike most of the population, some individuals may lack an enzyme required to metabolize a particular drug. Any unexpected reaction to a drug is commonly referred to as an idiosyncratic reaction, although the term may be more specifically used to define a genetically-determined abnormal response to a drug. Idiosyncratic reactions represent some of the most serious forms of adverse events since, by nature, they are unpredictable, and are not seen until the drug is administered. The identification of true idiosyncratic reactions is important in establishing the safety of medicines. In dentistry, most reported 'idiosyncratic' reactions to local anaesthetics are due to intravascular injection of the anaesthetic, or an anxiety reaction during injection.

Most of the time, individual variations to a drug will be seen as a difference in the magnitude of response (quantitative effect), although there can also be variations in the nature of the response too (qualitative effect). Such variations are normally seen between individuals, but may also happen within one individual on different occasions. These variations may be caused by a pharmacokinetic effect, where there is a difference in the concentration of the drug at the target site. However, one can also get a pharmacodynamic effect, where the concentration of the drug at the target site is the same, but the response to it differs. The main causes of these individual variations in drug response are the age of the patient, their genetic make-up, and drug–drug interactions.

Age

The influence of the patient's age mainly reflects differences in the renal excretion and hepatic metabolism of drugs, with both processes being less efficient in the very young, as well as the elderly. Unless drug doses are reduced appropriately, the reduced elimination of the drug may lead to increased, and potentially harmful, responses.

In the newborn, the rate of renal excretion is only about 20% of that in an adult, but by the end of the first week of life, full kidney function is established. The metabolic capacity of the liver is also limited, but assumes full adult function after the first two months. In the elderly, both renal and liver function decline. Kidney function starts to decline after 20 years of age, and by 75 years renal elimination may be half that of a young adult. Hepatic metabolism of drugs also declines slowly with age, but the rate of decline is more variable than that seen with renal function. It is also important to keep in mind that both renal and liver disease will also impact upon drug elimination.

Genetics

An individual's genetic make-up may have an important influence on drug responses, particularly as a result of altered metabolism. One will observe much less variation in responses between first-degree relatives, and very little between monozygotic (identical) twins. Most of the time, this variation follows a 'normal' distribution. However, in some cases, population may be divided into two distinct groups. For drugs whose hepatic metabolism relies on acetylation, such as the anti-tuberculosus drug, isoniazid, half of population are 'fast acetylators', which results in lower plasma concentrations of the drug, whilst the other half are 'slow acetylators', resulting in higher plasma concentrations. These metabolic differences are determined by a single gene.

Some individuals may lack specific metabolic enzyme activity, which may account not just for adverse responses, but also a lack of response to certain drugs. Suxamethonium is a drug used in anaesthesia to give a short-lasting paralysis of skeletal muscle (neuromuscular blocking agent). Normally its effects only last a few minutes because it is rapidly inactivated by the enzyme plasma cholinesterase. However, a few individuals lack this enzyme activity, and fail to inactivate suxamethonium. The resulting neuromuscular blockade can last for hours,

with potentially fatal consequences. Codeine, or methylmorphine, is a commonly used mild opioid analgesic agent for moderate pain. Codeine's analgesic effects rely on its conversion to morphine, a reaction catalysed by the hepatic enzyme, CYP2D6. Some individuals lack normal CYP2D6 metabolic activity, and as a result achieve little or no pain relief with codeine.

Drug–drug interactions

When appropriately managed, drug combinations can have beneficial effects, helping to increase treatment effectiveness or reduce side effects. On the other hand, drug combinations can also cause problems. For example, the side effects of multiple drugs may be additive, a problem seen when several drugs with CNS depressant activities are used in combination. Drug interactions can occur both as a result of pharmacodynamic and pharmacokinetic actions.

One patient group where drug interactions are likely to be more common is the elderly. More than half of elderly patients are taking five or more medications on a daily basis. While these medications may be indicated, this polypharmacy is not without its own risks.

Pharmacodynamic interactions

Pharmacodynamic interactions may be seen when two drugs that have either opposite effects, or similar effects, are co-administered. In terms of two drugs having opposite effects, one example would be the co-administration of a beta-blocker (beta-adrenoceptor antagonist) and a beta-adrenoceptor agonist. By blocking beta-adrenoceptors, albeit the β1-subtype, beta-blockers may reduce the effectiveness of bronchodilators, such as salbutamol.

In contrast, additive effects may be seen with drugs that have a similar pharmacodynamic action. Drugs that have an anxiolytic or sedative action, such as benzodiazepines, share one basic pharmacological characteristic, namely they are CNS depressants. While benzodiazepines produce a dose-dependent depression of the CNS, when used on their own they have a good safety margin. However, if they are taken in combination with alcohol, or other sedative agents, they can cause life-threatening respiratory depression. In this situation, the CNS depressant effects summate, potentially leading to respiratory depression and death.

Pharmacokinetic interactions

Pharmacokinetic interactions can affect all four phases of drug disposition (ADME), and may alter the concentration of the drug within the body, or at the target site.

Some interactions may affect the rate of drug absorption. For example, drugs that have an inhibitory effect on gastrointestinal motility, such as opioid analgesics, can slow the absorption of other drugs that are taken orally. However, this kind of interaction can be used to produce a clinical benefit too. Local anaesthetics are commonly formulated with a vasoconstrictor, such as adrenaline, in order to reduce local blood flow at the site of administration, thereby maintaining a higher concentration of anaesthetic at that site, and prolonging its action.

Drug interactions may also affect the distribution of drugs. These interactions are mainly due to competition for the binding sites on plasma proteins. Since binding site concentration is relatively high, and most drugs are administered at relatively low concentrations, it is not a common issue. However, there are a few drugs, including aspirin and drugs which are sulfonamides (antibiotics, diuretics, etc), which can displace other agents from plasma proteins. As a result, there is an increased free concentration of the displaced drug, potentially causing toxic reactions, but also increasing elimination. Drugs that alter the pH of selective body compartments may also affect drug distribution, but this impacts mainly on renal excretion.

Altered hepatic metabolism is a common reason for drug interactions. Many drugs, including ethanol, will induce hepatic enzymes, increasing their own metabolism, as well as that of other drugs. Increased drug metabolism can decrease the effectiveness of many treatments, including oral contraception, anticoagulant therapy, and epileptic medication. While enzyme induction mainly leads to the increased elimination of co-administered drugs, it can have more sinister consequences. If the enzyme induction leads to increased levels of toxic phase I metabolites, such as those associated with paracetamol, it can increase the toxic and carcinogenic effects of certain drugs.

Another common interaction with co-administered drugs is caused by competition between the drugs for the cytochrome enzymes. If one drug is able to compete more effectively, that can result in reduced metabolism of other drugs, resulting in higher, and potentially toxic levels of that drug. This competition can lead to dose-related toxic events, even although the dose of the individual drugs is 'correct'.

Interactions may also alter the excretion of drugs. As already mentioned, this may be influenced by changes in plasma protein binding, leading to increased free concentrations of one drug, and hence increased renal excretion. In the renal tubule there are carrier proteins that may play a role in tubular reabsorption or secretion. If two drugs are competing for the same carrier, this can lead to altered elimination, such as reduced secretion. This competition can be used to produce a clinical benefit. The drug probenecid will inhibit the tubular secretion of penicillin, and hence prolong its activity. Altering the pH of the glomerular filtrate in the kidney can also decrease the passive reabsorption of drugs by promoting ion trapping, hence increasing their elimination. Urinary acidifiers can increase the excretion of basic drugs, while urinary alkalinization will increase acidic drug elimination. Such approaches may be used to manage drug-overdose situations. Finally, diuretic drugs will increase urine output, and hence can increase the renal elimination of other drugs.

CHAPTER 4
Antimicrobials – antiseptics and disinfectants

Martina Shepard

Key Topics

- Overview of sterilisation, disinfection and antisepsis
- Antiseptics
  - Mouthwashes
  - Root canal treatment medicaments
  - Hand hygiene
- Disinfectants
  - Surface cleaning agents
  - Instrument cleaning agents
  - Impression and prosthesis disinfection
- Specific agents
  - Chlorhexidine
  - Iodophors
  - Triclosan
  - Alcohol
  - Quaternary ammonium compounds
  - Oxidising agents
  - Essential oils

Learning Objectives

- To understand the difference between sterilisation, disinfection and antisepsis
- To understand the mechanism of action of agents used for disinfection and antisepsis
- To be aware of the most effective agents for infection control in the dental surgery

Essential Dental Therapeutics, First Edition. Edited by David Wray.
© 2018 John Wiley & Sons Ltd. Published 2018 by John Wiley & Sons Ltd.
Companion Website: www.wiley.com/go/wray/dental-therapeutics

Introduction

Antiseptics and disinfectants are agents used to reduce the pathogenicity of microorganisms capable of causing infection. Antiseptics are used as medications in humans or animals, whereas disinfectants are used on inanimate objects or surfaces.

Antiseptics are commonly used in dentistry as mouthwashes, root canal medicaments, and hand hygiene products.

Disinfectants relevant to dental practice include those used to clean surfaces in the dental surgery and agents used for cleaning instruments.

It is important to understand the difference between the concepts of sterilization, disinfection and antisepsis. Sterilization implies the complete removal of all viable microorganisms, including viruses and spores. This requires the sustained application of high temperatures, chemicals and/or radiation. It is the highest level of cleansing that may be attained and is a requirement for the re-use of dental instruments, in order to prevent cross-infection in the dental practice setting.

Disinfection involves the use of chemicals to destroy the majority of pathogenic organisms on surfaces or objects. Disinfection leads to a reduction in pathogenicity but does not completely remove all microorganisms. It is not practical or possible to sterilize some objects in the dental surgery, such as benchtops, however it is well recognized that these objects do pose a risk of transmission of infection due to viable microorganisms being deposited on their surfaces via droplets, aerosols or direct contact from instruments or clinicians' hands and gloves. Disinfection is a key component in the prevention of cross-infection in the dental practice setting.

Antisepsis refers to the use of chemicals to reduce the number of pathogenic organisms on a living surface, such as skin or oral mucosa. Antisepsis may be used to prevent the development of infection, assist in management of an active infection or to prevent cross-infection.

The use of antiseptics and disinfectants will be considered in turn. This will be followed by a consideration of individual agents.

Table 4.1 Ideal properties of an antiseptic

- Active against a broad spectrum of pathogens, including bacteria, fungi, viruses and protozoa
- Cidal (killing) as well as static (limiting the growth of organisms)
- Capable of destroying spores
- Non-toxic and non-irritating to tissues
- Rapid onset and long duration of action
- Chemically stable, non-staining
- Acceptable smell and taste
- Active even in the presence of bodily oils, fluids, blood and other exudates
- Low cost

Antiseptics

The ideal qualities of an antiseptic are shown in Table 4.1.

Antisepsis in dentistry involves a variety of different indications. Hand hygiene is aimed at reducing the number of pathogenic organisms on the hands of dental clinical staff, as part of standard infection control precautions to reduce the risk of cross-infection.

The use of antiseptic mouthwashes is indicated for situations in which it is important to try to prevent infection, as well as part of treatment for an active infection. Antiseptic mouthwashes can form part of periodontal treatment as well as the management of other types of oral infective processes, including fungal and bacterial infections.

Concern has been raised about the high alcohol content of many mouthwashes and the possibility that this may be carcinogenic. Alcohol-free mouthwashes are widely available.

Antiseptic chemicals are often used as part of root canal treatment protocols, in order to reduce the number of viable bacteria in an infected root canal and reduce the risk of ongoing symptoms or infection.

The use of antiseptics in the oral cavity is affected by the presence of biofilms. Biofilms are an organized structure consisting of bacteria and extracellular material produced by bacteria, within which organisms may exist in a protected environment. This has implications for the efficacy of antiseptic agents as they may not be able to reach the most pathogenic bacteria, which exist deep within the biofilm. Various chemical properties of antiseptics have been trialled in an attempt to disrupt and penetrate biofilms for better antiseptic activity.

Mouthwashes

Mouthwashes used in dentistry include a variety of antiseptic agents, such as chlorhexidine, essential oils (menthol, thymol and eucalyptol) and cetylpyridinium chloride. Hydrogen peroxide is also available as a mouthwash.

Chlorhexidine:

Chlorhexidine is available in 0.12% and 0.2% mouthwash formulations, as well as a toothpaste and gel formula. Chlorhexidine mouthwash has excellent substantivity on the oral mucosa (up to 12 hours). It will inhibit the formation of plaque in a clean mouth, and as such is a useful adjunct to mechanical oral hygiene practices. It can also be useful in the symptomatic management of oral mucosal disorders.

Essential oils:

Essential oils are used in proprietary mouthwashes such as Listerine, and their antimicrobial activity is due to their ability to damage cell membranes, causing leakage of cell contents and cell lysis. They also inhibit bacterial enzymes and are able to penetrate biofilms and inhibit plaque formation. Some essential oils also have anti-inflammatory activity. The essential oils eucalyptol, thymol, methyl salicylate and menthol have been utilized in combination with alcohol as a mouthwash formulation.

Cetylpyridinium chloride:

Cetylpyridinium chloride is a quaternary ammonium compound used in some mouthwashes. Its mechanism of action is similar to chlorhexidine in that it is cationic and binds to bacterial cell membranes, causing membrane disruption and cell lysis.

Hydrogen peroxide:

Hydrogen peroxide produces free radicals which can attack microbial membranes, DNA and other cellular components. It has a wide spectrum of activity against fungi, bacteria, viruses and spores. Hydrogen peroxide 1.5% is available as a mouthwash and is particularly effective against anaerobic bacteria, due to the oxygen released as it degrades.

Root canal treatment medicaments

Sodium Hypochlorite:

Sodium hypochlorite (bleach) is commonly used as an irrigation agent during root canal therapy. It is toxic to living tissues and able to dissolve organic material. It will cause significant irritation if extruded beyond the apical area of the tooth.

Chlorhexidine:

Chlorhexidine has also been used as a root canal irrigant and in its gel form, as a root canal dressing.

Hand hygiene

Hand hygiene is an essential part of standard infection-control practices in healthcare. Hand hygiene reduces the transmission of microorganisms between healthcare professionals (HCP) and patients, reducing the risk of infection acquisition in healthcare settings by both patients and HCPs. WHO guidance suggests that hand hygiene practices should be employed in the following '5 moments':

1. Before patient contact
2. Before aseptic tasks
3. After exposure to a body fluid
4. After patient contact
5. After contact with the patient environment

Hand hygiene procedures include handwashing with soap and water, and the use of hand cleansing rubs. Hand hygiene is essential even when procedures are carried out wearing gloves. It is suggested that all members of a dental practice have regularly updated training in hand hygiene procedures and that signage (such as that available from the WHO) is placed around the practice as an *aide memoir*.

A more specific description of required moments for hand hygiene in dental practice is listed in the UK Health and Technical Memorandum 05-01, as shown in Table 4.2.

Hand hygiene using soap and water requires a standardized washing technique lasting for 40–60 seconds in order to achieve the maximal reduction in viable microorganisms on the hands. In order to clean hands and wrists most effectively, sleeves should be rolled up above the elbow, watches, jewellery and rings should be removed, and nail varnish should not be worn.

Antiseptic agents used for handwashing include chlorhexidine gluconate, povidone-iodine and triclosan.

Handrubs were introduced as an alternative method of hand hygiene in healthcare settings, and are now considered equivalent or even superior to handwashing as a method of preventing healthcare acquired infections. Alcohol-based handrubs have a broader antimicrobial spectrum than most handwashing agents, and the technique is preferable in many ways, as it is more quickly undertaken, more easily accessible than techniques requiring water, and better tolerated by the skin. Handrub solutions can be made available at the patient's bedside and in all settings requiring hand hygiene procedures, due to the convenient pump-pack dispensers. This may also increase compliance with hand hygiene procedures due to the ease of access to the handrubs, and the shorter time required for decontamination.

WHO guidance for hand hygiene using alcohol-based handrubs advises that the procedure should last for 20–30 seconds, and all surfaces must be covered equally.

Agents used as handrubs include alcohol either alone or in combination with chlorhexidine gluconate.

Disinfectants

The ideal properties of a disinfectant are shown in Table 4.3.

Microbes have differing levels of resistance to disinfection agents. Bacterial spores are the most resistant microbe. The spore coat is resistant to most environmental challenges and the microbe remains viable, but dormant, inside the spore. In the right conditions it will germinate and form an active and infectious organism. Generally, only oxidizing agents are sufficiently potent to inactivate spores.

Mycobacteria have a waxy external coat which makes them relatively resistant to disinfectants. Disinfectants labelled 'tuberculocidal' are able to

Table 4.2 Hand hygiene in dental practice
1. Before and after treatment
2. Before and after the removal of personal protective equipment (mask, eye protection, aprons, gowns, gloves etc.)
3. After washing contaminated instruments
4. Before touching clean/sterilized instruments
5. After decontamination of instruments or surfaces
6. After contact with devices used for decontamination

Table 4.3 The ideal properties of a disinfectant
• Active against a broad spectrum of pathogens, including bacteria, fungi, viruses and protozoa
• Cidal (killing) as well as static (limiting the growth of organisms), capable of destroying spores
• Non-corrosive to surfaces/instruments
• Rapid action and long duration of action
• Chemically stable, non-staining
• Low odour and non-irritating to skin/eyes/airways
• Easily removed by washing

inactivate these bacteria and are generally required for hospital-level disinfection.

Non-enveloped viruses such as norovirus and rotavirus are also resistant to most disinfectant agents. These viruses lack a lipid capsule, and the viral capsid is resistant to alcohol as well as lipophilic disinfectants such as quaternary ammonium compounds.

Disinfection is an essential part of standard infection control in dental practice, as there are a variety of sources of potential infection for both dental care professionals and patients. These include contaminated instruments, surfaces, impression materials, prosthetics and waterlines.

Dental unit waterlines (DUWL) form a particular problem in that they support the development of biofilms. Biofilms may be resistant to standard decontamination procedures due to their organized structure, which can protect pathogenic organisms and reduce the access of disinfectant chemicals to the organisms at the base of the biofilm.

Surface cleaning agents

Surface cleaning is an essential part of infection control in dental practices. Due to the use of high speed drills with water irrigation, ultrasonic scalers, rotary polishers and the use of these devices in the presence of saliva, the generation of aerosols containing infective microorganisms is a common situation in dental practice. Aerosols may be deposited on any surfaces within the dental surgery. Spatter from procedures or direct contact by a contaminated instrument or gloves are other means whereby infective material may become present on a surface.

The ideal surface cleaning agent is active against bacteria, fungi and viruses. It should be able to inactivate hepatitis and HIV viruses. Higher-grade disinfectants are also tuberculocidal.

Surface cleansing should not be done with reusable cloths as these harbour microorganisms. Pre-saturated wipes or single use cloths should be used to clean surfaces.

The majority of pre-saturated wipes or disinfectant agents used for surface cleansing in dental surgeries contain alcohol, quaternary ammonium compounds, or a combination of these. They may also contain chlorines or hydrogen peroxide.

Surfaces heavily contaminated with blood should be cleaned with an appropriate agent (such as a chlorine-containing solution), as alcohol-based surface cleansing agents are less effective in the presence of protein.

Instrument cleaning agents

Disinfection of instruments is used as an adjunct to heat sterilization for instruments that come into contact with the tissues or bodily fluids.

It is important that disinfectants or detergents specifically designed for instrument cleaning are used for this purpose. Alcohol and chlorhexidine cause protein in biological material to adhere to metal instruments, which may lead to residue remaining on the instruments prior to sterilization. This can lead to the retention of potentially infectious organisms on the instruments, even after sterilization.

Chemical disinfection with commonly available agents is not considered an alternative to heat sterilization for instruments that have been used in operative dentistry.

Impression and prosthesis disinfection

Prior to transport to the laboratory, impressions and prostheses that have been in contact with the patient's oral cavity need to be disinfected. It is important that appropriate disinfectant agents are used in order to avoid damaging the impression or prosthetic material. The majority of impression material manufacturers will give instructions regarding appropriate agents for disinfection, and proprietary disinfectants are available for this purpose.

Specific agents

Chlorhexidine

Chlorhexidine is a cationic bisbiguanide. Its mechanism of action relies on its ability to bind to and disrupt cell membranes, due to its strongly cationic nature. It has good substantivity as it will bind to biological surfaces and remain active for up to 12 hours. It has a broad spectrum of activity against bacterial, viral and fungal organisms. It is bacteriostatic at low concentrations and bactericidal at high concentrations.

Chlorhexidine is widely used in medicine and dentistry. It is used for hand antisepsis including as a surgical scrub solution, and as a component of alcohol-based hand rubs used in healthcare settings. Solutions containing a combination of alcohol and chlorhexidine have long-lasting antimicrobial activity.

Applications in dentistry include the use of chlorhexidine-containing mouthwashes, dentifrices, gels, slow-release periodontal 'chips' and as root canal irrigants.

Chlorhexidine is incompatible with anionic components found in most toothpastes and antifungal treatments such as Nystatin, and should be used at a different time to these agents (for example, half an hour later).

Chlorhexidine has demonstrated anti-plaque activity, and this is mainly due to its excellent substantivity (ability to bind to surfaces and remain active). It is active against a variety of bacteria in dental plaque, and it can reduce salivary bacterial counts by up to 80% after a single mouthrinse. Chlorhexidine binds to mucins in the salivary pellicle and inhibits bacterial colonization.

Use of chlorhexidine-containing mouthrinse or gel leads to a significant reduction in plaque levels and gingival inflammation, and it is frequently used as an adjunct in the management of gingivitis and periodontitis. It is particularly useful in situations where optimal oral hygiene procedures cannot be carried out, such as in patients with medical conditions or disabilities preventing adequate plaque control.

Chlorhexidine leads to a reduction in Streptococcus mutans counts in plaque and saliva. Consequently, the use of chlorhexidine-containing varnishes has been suggested as a means of dental caries prevention. However recent reviews of studies in this field have found that the evidence to support this practice is poor.

Chlorhexidine may be used as anti-candidal therapy, both for management of mild mucosal candidal infection and for cleaning of removable partial dentures. Dentures may be soaked in chlorhexidine periodically to maintain low candidal levels, and alternate day rinsing with chlorhexidine mouthwash can be helpful in the management of mild candidal infections, or as prophylaxis in patients with risk factors for recurrent candidiasis.

Chlorhexidine is used in the management of patients suffering from acute mucositis secondary to chemotherapy and/or radiotherapy. It forms part of the standard oral care regimen for patients undergoing conditioning prior to stem cell transplantation. Chlorhexidine is available in an alcohol-free formulation.

Chlorhexidine causes extrinsic staining of dental surfaces and the dorsum of the tongue. The extrinsic staining of the teeth is due to binding of chromogenic foodstuffs such as red wine or coffee and tea. This is more of a problem with the 0.2% mouthwash. These changes are temporary and the staining can be removed by professional hygiene procedures. Chlorhexidine may also lead to dysgeusia (taste abnormality) in some patients. Rarely mucosal sluffing may occur as a hypersensitivity reaction.

It is also important that dental practitioners are aware of reports of anaphylactic reactions to chlorhexidine, including the use of chlorhexidine-containing mouthwashes. The majority of these cases relate to the use of chlorhexidine-coated central venous catheters, or the topical application of chlorhexidine-containing solutions to the urogenital mucosa. However there have been some reports of fatal anaphylaxis secondary to the use of chlorhexidine in the oral cavity, and it is important for all dental care professionals to take a thorough allergy history prior to prescribing or using products containing chlorhexidine.

Iodophors

Iodophors consist of iodine complexed to a water-soluble carrier molecule. Their antimicrobial action is due to the release of free iodine, which is a highly active microbicidal agent against bacteria, spores, fungi and viruses. The antimicrobial action of iodine is due to its effects on protein and nucleic acid structure and synthesis.

Povidone-iodine is an example of an iodophor commonly used as an antiseptic agent. It has a broad spectrum of activity, particularly against skin organisms, and it is often used as a surgical hand scrub.

Iodophors may also be used as disinfectant agents, with tuberculocidal, fungicidal, virucidal, and bactericidal activity. The majority of commercially available iodophors are not active against spores.

Iodophors may discolour some surfaces, and it is important to avoid their use in patients with an iodine allergy.

Triclosan

Triclosan's antimicrobial activity is due to its effect on fatty acid synthesis, which makes it bacteriostatic at low concentrations. At higher concentrations it is bactericidal, and this is thought to be due to cell membrane damage. It has antibacterial activity as well as some antifungal activity.

Triclosan is present in a variety of household products such as antimicrobial soaps and deodorants. It is also present in mouthwashes and toothpastes. In healthcare settings triclosan is used as a handwashing agent and as a surgical scrub.

Alcohol

Ethyl alcohol and isopropyl alcohol are used as disinfectant agents in the healthcare setting. The antimicrobial activity of alcohol relates to its ability to denature microbial proteins. Alcohol is bactericidal at concentrations above 50% and the optimal concentration to achieve maximal bactericidal, tuberculocidal, fungicidal and virucidal activity is between 60 and 90%. Alcohol is not sporicidal and its antimicrobial activity is reduced in the presence of large amounts of protein. This makes it ineffective as a disinfection agent when items are heavily contaminated with blood or other body fluids.

Alcohol can damage the surfaces of some materials, and it evaporates quickly so ensuring adequate contact time for microbicidal activity can be difficult. Alcohol can be irritating and dehydrating to skin and other tissues in high concentrations.

Quaternary ammonium compounds

Quaternary ammonium compounds are used in healthcare settings as surface disinfection agents. Their antimicrobical action is due to denaturation of cell proteins, cell membrane disruption and enzyme inactivation. They are microbicidal, virucidal and fungicidal, but are not active against tuberculosis, non-enveloped viruses or spores.

Quaternary ammonium compounds are often used in combination with alcohol, chlorines and/or phenols as pre-saturated disinfectant wipes.

Quaternary ammonium compounds may also be used as antiseptics, for example in mouthwashes, soaps and shampoos. Cetylpyridinium chloride is a quaternary ammonium compound commonly present in mouthwashes and toothpastes. It has anti-plaque activity and is an effective adjunct to oral hygiene procedures for reducing the severity of gingivitis. It may also be useful as an anti-halitosis product.

Oxidizing agents

Oxidizing agents damage microbial cell membranes and cause cell lysis, as well as producing free radicals that damage DNA.

Oxidizing agents used in dentistry include sodium hypochlorite and hydrogen peroxide. These may be used as disinfectants, such as for disinfection of impression materials, or for surface cleaning.

These agents are also used as antiseptics. Hydrogen peroxide mouthwash may be used for the management of anaerobic infections such as acute necrotizing ulcerative gingivitis. Sodium hypochlorite is commonly used as a root canal irrigant during endodontic therapy.

Essential oils

Essential oils consist of a mixture of volatile chemicals produced by plants as metabolic by-products. Their antimicrobial activity is due to their ability to damage cell membranes, causing leakage of cell contents and cell lysis. They also inhibit bacterial enzymes, damage DNA and are able to penetrate biofilms.

Essential oils that have been employed in healthcare settings include tea tree oil (from *Melaleuca alternifolia*), thymol and carvacrol (from thyme and oregano), clove oil (from *Syzygium aromaticum*) and eucalyptus oil.

There is some evidence that essential oil-containing mouthwashes may be beneficial as an adjunct to oral hygiene procedures for the management of gingivitis.

CHAPTER 5

Antimicrobials – antibiotics

Esther Hullah

Key Topics

- Overview
- Choice of antibiotic
- Mechanism of action of antibiotics
- Pharmacokinetics
- Antibiotic prophylaxis

Learning Objectives

- To be aware of the importance of the correct choice of antibiotic in different circumstances
- To understand the issues around antibiotic prophylaxis in dentistry

Essential Dental Therapeutics, First Edition. Edited by David Wray.
© 2018 John Wiley & Sons Ltd. Published 2018 by John Wiley & Sons Ltd.
Companion Website: www.wiley.com/go/wray/dental-therapeutics

Introduction

An antibiotic is defined as a substance produced by, or derived from, a microorganism that destroys or inhibits the growth of other microorganisms. Antibiotics aim to be selectively toxic to the invading bacteria while having minimal effect on the host.

The discovery of antibiotics transformed the management and outcomes of bacterial infections and facilitated the ability to safely perform surgical procedures. This pivotal advance in therapeutics was quickly eroded by the emergence of antibiotic resistance, especially by staphylococci, and antimicrobial resistance to antibiotics threatens to become the major global health challenge of the century. Antibiotic prescribing stewardship is now of utmost importance to good clinical practice among prescribers of whom dental practitioners form a significant part.

Dentists are the second largest group of prescribers of antibiotics to patients after medical practitioners and antibiotics are by far the largest group of drugs prescribed by dentists who prescribe antibiotics on almost a daily basis. A proper understanding of the rationale underpinning the appropriate prescription of antibiotics in dental practice is therefore of paramount importance not only to provide optimal clinical care but also to protect society from the devastating consequences of increasing antimicrobial resistance to drugs.

Antibiotics may be appropriately prescribed to treat uncontrolled infection or may be used prophylactically to prevent infection. These uses of antibiotics will now be considered in turn followed by a discussion of both patient and microbial factors, which are important when prescribing antibiotics. Finally, there will be a consideration of the individual groups of available antibiotics.

Management of infection

Bacterial infections of the mouth may arise from dental infection causing apical abscess formation or from infection of the periodontium or gingivae including pericoronitis. Less commonly, bacterial mucosal infections or sinusitis may occur.

Antibiotics are indicated to treat infections where there is evidence of spreading infection such as cellulitis, lymph node involvement, local swelling or evidence of systemic involvement such as pyrexia, malaise or leucocytosis.

Specifically, there is no evidence to support the use of antibiotics in alveolar osteitis (dry socket) or pulpitis which do not meet the criteria for prescribing antibiotics.

Dental abscesses are usually infected with *viridans Streptococci spp.* or Gram negative organisms or both. These organisms are usually susceptible to penicillin antibiotics. Although best practice suggests antibiotics should be prescribed with knowledge of the sensitivities of the infecting organism, in primary-care dental practice, antibiotics are usually prescribed empirically and, for the above reasons, penicillins are usually appropriate and effective.

The use of broad spectrum antibiotics encourages the emergence of *Clostridium difficile*-associated disease, especially in vulnerable groups and those on proton pump inhibitors and so should be avoided. Similarly, broad spectrum drugs encourage the emergence of resistant forms of *Staphylococci spp.* which has negative public health implications and should be avoided as first line drugs.

Patients who have received an antibiotic within the last six weeks are at risk of harbouring resistant organisms, however, and so a different antibiotic should be prescribed on the second occasion.

Dental abscess

Antibiotics are not appropriate for the management of localized periapical infection even in the presence of localized swelling. Treatment, in the first instance, should be by drainage of the abscess either by extraction or through the root canal. Fluctuant swellings should be incised to allow drainage although this should not be performed if there is evidence of cellulitis. Antibiotics should only be prescribed if there is evidence of spreading infection as outlined above.

Floor of mouth swelling, difficulty breathing or trismus suggests infection of tissue spaces and is an emergency requiring admission to hospital.

Patients given antibiotics should be reviewed after 24 to 48 hours to assess any improvement. A lack of clinical response may indicate microbial resistance and the need for alternative antibiotic medication.

Antibiotic therapy should continue until a clinical response indicates that the immune system is, once again, coping with the infection, usually five days. Antibiotic courses should not be prolonged since this encourages the development of antibiotic resistance.

Necrotizing ulcerative gingivitis and pericoronitis

Necrotizing ulcerative gingivitis is an anaerobic fuso-spirocaetal bacterial infection of the gingival margins which is usually localized and can be managed by local measures. More severe cases or those with evidence of spreading infection should also be given antibiotics.

Pericoronitis is also an anaerobic infection around an erupting tooth and can usually be managed by local measures. Again, evidence of spreading infection is an indication for antibiotics.

For both necrotizing ulcerative gingivitis and pericoronitis, which are anaerobic infections, metronidazole is the drug of first choice although amoxicillin is also effective.

Oral mucosal infections

Bacterial infections affecting the oral mucosa are rare and should be treated either with topical antiseptics or with antibiotics with appropriate knowledge of the infecting organism and its sensitivities.

Sinusitis

Sinusitis is usually self-limiting and responds to steam inhalations. Persistent or purulent sinusitis should respond to a penicillin antibiotic such as amoxicillin.

Periodontal disease

Antibiotics may be used in specialist periodontal practice as an adjunct in periodontal therapy to control acute episodes of periodontitis. Therapy usually uses metronidazole or a tetracycline or amoxicillin.

Antibiotic prophylaxis

Antibiotic prophylaxis may be used for surgical prophylaxis such as before colonic or prostatic surgery or it may be prescribed to prevent infective endocarditis after dental procedures.

Surgical prophylaxis is not required for oral surgical procedures and there is no evidence it confers any advantages.

Historically, antibiotic prophylaxis for infective endocarditis was recommended for patients at increased risk of developing endocarditis as a result of bacteraemias arising from dental procedures. In 2008, the National Institute for Health and Clinical Excellence (NICE) issued Clinical Guidance 64 (www.nice.org.uk/guidance/cg64). This stated that antibiotic prophylaxis was not recommended before dental procedures. This was concluded in light of a lack of evidence for the efficacy of antibiotics used prophylactically for prevention. Also there was evidence that everyday activities such as tooth brushing gave rise to bacteraemias without dental procedures. Furthermore, oral hygiene was felt to be importance in the prevention of endocarditis and that antibiotic prophylaxis regimes may act as a barrier to best oral hygiene regimes. Finally, the risks of antibiotic prophylaxis may outweigh the benefits.

Such a paradigm shift in thinking around accepted prophylactic regimes has caused a significant dichotomy of opinion especially between cardiologists and the dental profession and is perpetuated by opposite advice from Europe and the United States. NICE guidance remains extant, however, and advice within the current British National Formulary reflects this.

Prescribing considerations

Notwithstanding the considerations above regarding the specific management of oral infections there are a number of overarching factors that influence the choice of antibiotic. Before choosing an antibiotic the clinician must consider two factors – the patient and the known or causative organism.

The patient

Several patient-orientated factors should be taken into account before prescribing antibiotics. The patient's age, sex, weight and general state of health must be considered when choosing both the drug and its dose.

Documentation of infection:

Whenever possible, clinical suspicion of infection should be supported by laboratory diagnosis. Relevant samples, for example sputum, urine, pus, blood should be obtained before treatment is commenced.

Age:

Drug kinetics are influenced by age-dependent changes in the path of elimination.

Renal and hepatic function:

Many commonly used antimicrobials are eliminated by the kidney while a few undergo hepatic metabolism. Dose modification is likely to be necessary if renal function is moderately or severely impaired. Drug monitoring is mandatory for antimicrobials with concentration-related toxicity (see Table 5.1).

Drug sensitivity:

Previous exposure to drugs should always be asked about. Penicillins and cephalosporins are the antimicrobials most frequently associated with sensitivity reactions and there is a 5–10% cross-sensitivity between these two drug groups because they both contain a β-lactam ring. Sulphonamides also frequently cause allergic reactions.

Diminished resistance in infection:

Patients with malignant disease, HIV or who are receiving cytotoxic or immunosuppressant drugs are susceptible to severe infections often with less common organisms, for example commensal bacteria, some viruses, yeasts, fungi and protozoa.

Pregnancy:

Penicillins and cephalosporins are not harmful to the foetus. Foetal damage has been associated definitely with streptomycin and tetracyclines. Possible adverse fetal effects have been ascribed to gentamicin and co-trimoxazole.

Antibiotics and contraception:

Previously broad-spectrum antibiotics were thought to reduce the efficacy of oral contraceptives. It is now recognized that antibiotics that do not induce liver enzymes do not cause this problem. In a dental practice environment this is not, therefore, important and additional contraceptive measures are not required unless the prescribed antibiotic causes diarrhoea or vomiting which might interfere with oral contraceptive absorption.

Microbiological considerations

Microbial factors such as sensitivity and resistance must be considered when prescribing an antibiotic.

Sensitivity

Bactericidal drugs destroy the organism against which they are effective. Bacteriostatic drugs do not kill the organism but destroy its ability to replicate.

Table 5.1 Antimicrobials for which dose modification is required in mild, moderate or severe renal failure and in liver disease

Renal failure			
Mild	**Moderate**	**Severe**	**Liver disease**
Aminglycosides	Metronidazole	Co-trimoxazole	Clindamycin
Cephalosporins	Ticarcillin	Penicillins	Isoniazid
Ethambutol		Acyclovir	Rifampicin
Flucytosine			
Vancomycin			
Avoid: Cephalothin, Nitrofurantoin, tetracyclines			*Avoid*: Erythromycin

The known or likely organism and its antibacterial sensitivity, in association the above factors, will suggest one or more antibacterials.

Resistance

Some bacteria have always been resistant to the effects of certain drugs, while others have developed resistance in the course of repeated exposure to antimicrobials.

General aspects of antibiotic drugs

There are a number of general aspects of antibiotics that need to be elucidated such as absorption, tissue distribution and so on.

Absorption

Certain antimicrobials, for example aminoglycosides can only be given parenterally because absorption from the gastrointestinal tract is negligible. The decision on a drug formulation depends on the severity of the illness and the need to achieve high tissue concentrations.

Tissue distribution

General consideration of tissue distribution not only includes blood concentration, protein binding and lipid solubility but also the presence of inflammation, which tends to improve tissue penetration.

Route of elimination

This is usually by renal or hepatic metabolism.

Adverse effects

These are of two general types:

Hypersensitivity reactions:

Hypersensitivity reactions are either immediate or delayed. Immediate hypersensitivity produces anaphylaxis while delayed hypersensitivity commonly manifests as a rash. Hypersensitivity reactions usually occur without prior warning and are most commonly seen with penicillins, cephalosporins and sulphonamides.

Adverse reactions:

Adverse reaction can also be dose related, for example aminoglycosides and ototoxicity. Fortunately, the toxic concentrations of most antimicrobials in common use greatly exceed the required therapeutic concentrations. When this is not the case, for example gentamicin, drug level monitoring is mandatory.

Drug interactions

These can be either kinetic, for example enzyme inhibition or induction or dynamic, for example two drugs adversely affecting the same organ. It is important to check all interactions in an up to date formulary.

Mechanisms of action

Drugs that inhibit cell wall synthesis

This group includes penicillins, cephalosporins and vancomycin.

Bacterial cells have a unique peptidoglycan cell wall and thus drugs that act here do not affect eukaryotic cells. The penicillins and cephalosporins both contain a β-lactam ring within their structure. They produce their antimicrobial action by preventing cross-linkage between the linear peptidoglycan polymer chains that make up the cell wall. The growing bacteria become unable to maintain an osmotic gradient and swell and rupture. Their actions are bactericidal. Resistance to penicillins and cephalosporins may occur due to the production of β-lactamase enzymes by many bacteria, which inactivate the drugs. Structurally, the cephalosporins possess a dihydrothiazine ring connected to the β-lactam ring that makes them more resistant to hydrolysis by β-lactamases than the penicillins. There is, however, increasing concern regarding their use and the spread of *Clostridium difficile*.

Drugs that inhibit protein synthesis

Aminoglycosides, tetracyclines, chloramphenicol, macrolides and fusidic acid are included in this group.

Bacterial ribosomes have 50S and 30S units (S = Svedberg) compared with mammalian ribosomes, which have 60S and 40S subunits. Drugs can exploit this difference. Although the exact mechanism of action of the above drugs differs slightly, they all act to inhibit bacterial protein synthesis.

Aminoglycosides:

Gentamicin, streptomycin and neomycin bind irreversibly to the 30S portion of the bacterial ribosome. This inhibits the translation of m-RNA to protein and also causes the incorrect reading of the code on the m-RNA. They are bactericidal.

Tetracyclines:

Doxycycline and minocycline bind reversibly to the 30S subunit of the bacterial ribosome and interfere with the attachment of the t-RNA to the m-RNA ribosome complex. They are bacteriostatic.

Chloramphenicol:

Chloramphenicol binds reversibly to the 50S portion of the bacterial ribosome inhibiting the formation of peptide bonds. They can be bactericidal or bacteriostatic depending on the bacterial species.

Macrolides:

Erythromycin binds irreversibly to the 50S subunit of the bacterial ribosome preventing translocation movement of the ribosome along the m-RNA. They can be bactericidal or bacteriostatic depending on the bacterial species.

Fusidic acid:

Fusidic acid is a steroid that prevents binding of t-RNA to the ribosome.

Drugs that inhibit nucleic acid synthesis

This group includes antifolates, quinolones and rifampicin.

The bacterial genome is in the form of a single circular strand of DNA plus plamids (sometimes) which are not enclosed by a nuclear envelope (compared with eukaryotic chromosome arrangement within the nucleus). Drugs may thus interfere directly or indirectly with microbial DNA or RNA metabolism, replication and transcription.

Antifolates:

These drugs include sulphonamides, trimethoprim and co-trimoxazole. Folates are essential co-factors in the synthesis of purines and pyrimidines and thus of DNA. Unlike mammalian cells, which take up folate supplied in the diet, bacteria must synthesize their own folate which they do from para-aminobenzoic acid.

Quinolones:

Ciprofloxacin and nalidixic acid inhibit DNA-gyrase, the enzyme that compresses bacterial DNA into supercoils and is essential for the DNA replication and repair. They are bactericidal.

Other important drugs

Metronidazole:

This is a bactericidal drug that is metabolized within bacterial cells to a toxic intermediate that inhibits bacterial DNA synthesis and degrades existing bacterial DNA.

Pharmacokinetics

The pharmacokinetics of the various groups of antibiotics are discussed in the following subsections.

Penicillins

Absorption:

Penicillins have varied oral absorption. They are destroyed to some extent by gastric acid and therefore should be given on an empty stomach.

Distribution:

Penicillins have good penetration into most tissues.

Elimination:

Penicillins undergo enterohepatic circulation. The major route of elimination after reabsorption is active secretion in the renal tubules. Dose modification is required in severe renal failure.

Adverse effects:

Immediate hypersensitivity occurs in 0.05% of patients. Delayed hypersensitivity occurs in less than 5% of patients.

Drug interactions:

The anticoagulant effect of warfarin is potentiated by amoxicillin.

Antibacterial spectrum:

Certain organisms produce β-lactamase enzymes, which destroy the β-lactam ring of the penicillin molecule. Amoxycillin may be combined with clavulanic acid, which itself has no antibacterial activity but inhibits β-lactamase.

Penicillinase-sensitive penicillins:

Benzylpenicillin and phenoxypenicillins are active against *streptococci*, *pneumococci*, *gonococci* and *meningococci*. Ampicillin is broader spectrum and effective against some strains of *Escherichia coli*, *Proteus mirabilis*, *Shigella*, *Salmonella*, *Haemophilus influenza* and various *enterococci*. Amoxycillin is a better absorber derivative of Ampicillin.

Penicillinase-resistant penicillins:

Flucloxacillin is indicated in the treatment of infections caused by penicillinase producing *staphylococci*.

Cephalosporins

Absorption:

Cephalosporins are effective orally and distribute widely. They are eliminated renally.

Adverse effects:

Hypersensitivity is the main adverse effect, with around a 10% cross-reactivity with penicillin-sensitive patients.

Antibacterial spectrum:

The early cephalosporins were broad based but with limited activity against Gram-negative organisms. Cephamandole and cefuroxime are more resistant to β-lactamases and are more effective against a number of Gram-negative bacilli.

Other β-lactam antibiotics

These include Aztreonam, Imipenem, Meropenem and Ertapenem.

Aztreonam is a moncyclic β-lactam with an antibacterial spectrum limited to Gram-negative aerobic bacteria including *Pseudomonas aeruginosa*, *Neisseria meningitides* and *Haemophilus influenza*. Imipenem, a carbapenem, has a broad spectrum of activity including many aerobic and anaerobic Gram-positive and Gram-negative bacteria. It is co-administered with enzyme inhibitor Cilastatin as it is inactivated by renal enzymes. Meropenem is similar to Imipenem but is not inactivated by renal enzymes and therefore can be given without Cilastatin. Ertampenem has a broad spectrum that covers Gram-positive and Gram-negative organism and anaerobes. It is licensed for treating abdominal and gynaecological infections and for community-acquired pneumonia.

Aminoglycosides

Absorption:

Oral absorption of aminoglycosides is negligible. Elimination is by glomerular filtration.

Adverse effects:

Dose-related nephrotoxicity and ototoxicity can occur.

Drug interactions:

Nephrotoxicity is enhanced by co-administration with cephaloridine or polymixin. Ototoxicity is enhanced by loop diuretics.

Antibacterial spectrum:

Gentamicin is the most widely used aminoglycoside and is active against all aerobic Gram-negative rods, including *pseudomonas* and *proteus* and also against *staphylococci*.

Sulphonamide-trimethoprim combinations

Co-trimoxazole contains a sulphonamide, sulphamethoxazole and trimethoprim in a 5:1 ratio.

Absorption:

Co-trimoxazole is well absorbed orally and is also available for intravenous use. It is widely distributed and renally excreted.

Adverse effects:

Sulphonamides can cause rashes and much less commonly Steven-Johnson syndrome, renal failure and blood dyscrasias. Trimethoprim has been implicated in teratogenesis.

Drug interactions:

They can decrease the clearance of phenytoin, tolbutamide and warfarin. Displacement of methotrexate from protein binding sites can also lead to toxicity.

Antibacterial spectrum:

These are broad spectrum drugs.

Tetracyclines

Absorption:

Tetracyclines are absorbed orally. Tissue distribution is good and they are eliminated mainly unmetabolized by biliary excretion.

Adverse effects:

Tetracyclines bind to calcium in bones and teeth, leading to impaired bone growth and discoloration of teeth during active metabolism. They cross the placenta and are contraindicated in pregnancy and in children.

Drug interactions:

Milk, antacids, calcium, magnesium and iron form insoluble complexes with tetracyclines in the gut lumen leading to treatment failure.

Antibacterial spectrum:

They are active against a wide range of bacteria but resistance is increasing.

Quinolones

Nalidixic acid:

Nalidixic acid, the first quinolone, has been available for 30 years. It is administered orally and is used for uncomplicated urinary tract infections. Chemical modifications have produced a series of improved drugs and the most recent 4-fluoroquinolones; ciprofloxacin is the first agent in this group available in the UK.

Ciprofloxacin:

Ciprofloxacin is bactericidal and acts by interfering with DNA replication. It is well absorbed after oral administration and is distributed widely. Most of the drug is eliminated unaltered by the kidneys; the remainder is excreted by hepatic metabolism or unchanged in the faeces. Adverse effects are usually minor and include gastrointestinal upset. It is contraindicated in children and growing adolescents as it can cause damage to cartilage. Its absorption is reduced by the co-administration of aluminium and magnesium antacids. It interferes with the metabolism of theophylline, caffeine and warfarin. It is broad spectrum.

Other antibacterial drugs

Metronidazole:

Metronidazole is effective again anaerobic bacteria. The only major adverse effects are peripheral neuropathy following prolonged therapy and seizures following high doses. It is contra-indicated in pregnancy. It is an antimicrobial rather than an antibiotic since it is not a bacterial product.

Erythromycin:

Erythromycin has an antibacterial spectrum similar to penicillin and is a suitable second line drug for penicillin-allergic patients. It is bacteriostatic. It is associated with a high prevalence of nausea. The only major adverse effect is cholestatic jaundice and it is therefore contraindicated in liver disease.

Chloramphenicol:

Chloramphenicol is a very effective broad spectrum bacteriostatic antibiotic but its use is restricted because of bone marrow suppression, which can occur as a rare complication of treatment.

Fusidic acid:

Fusidic acid is narrow spectrum and is indicated in combination with another anti-staphylococal drug only in serious penicillin-resistant *staphylococci* infections. It is available as a cream for the treatment of staphylococcal skin infections including angular cheilitis.

Clindamycin:

Clindamycin is effective against penicillin-resistant *staphylococci* and many anaerobic organisms. A major adverse effect is pseudomembranous colitis caused by a toxin produced by *Clostridium difficile*.

Nitrofurantoin:

Nitrofurantoin is oral administered and achieves antibacterial concentrations only in urine and is effective against many organisms infecting the urinary tract. It has frequent adverse effects including gastrointestinal symptoms and rashes.

Vancomycin and Teicoplanin:

Vancomycin and teicoplanin are effective against *Clostridium difficile* and can be given orally to treat pseudomembranous colitis.

Tuberculosis

Tuberculosis (TB) is a disease caused by *Mycobacterium tuberculosis*. It usually affects the lungs, known as pulmonary TB, however it can be extrapulmonary (e.g. affecting lymph glands) or latent TB, where a patient has been infected with the mycobacterium but does not have any active signs of the disease.

Patients are most at risk of developing active TB if they are immunocompromised, such as following an organ transplant or on treatment for conditions such as cancer or rheumatoid arthritis.

The most common symptoms are a productive cough with blood stained sputum, weight loss, reduced appetite and fever with sweating particularly at night.

Principles of treatment

TB can usually be completely cured if medication is taken for at least 6 months. It is very important patients complete the full course of antibiotics. Drug administration needs to be fully supervised (directly observed therapy, DOT) in patients who cannot fully comply reliably with the treatment regime.

Immunocompromised patients

Multi-resistant TB maybe present in immunocompromised patients. The organism should always be cultured to confirm its type and drug sensitivity.

Specialist advice should be sought about TB treatment or chemoprophylaxis in HIV-positive individuals and care is required in choosing the regime and in avoiding potentially hazardous interactions. Starting antiretroviral treatment in the first 2 months of TB treatment increases the risk of immune reconstitution syndrome.

Infection maybe caused by other mycobacteri, for example the *M avium* complex in which specialist advice on management is needed.

Prevention of TB:

Some individuals develop TB due to reactivation of previously latent disease and chemoprophylaxis maybe required.

Treatment of pulmonary TB

Isoniazid and Rifampicin for 6 months with additional Pyrazinamide and Ethambutol for the first 2 months.

Extrapulmonary TB

The same combination is used as those to treat pulmonary TB however the drugs may need to be taken for 12 months.

Latent TB:

Treatment for latent TB is generally recommended for anyone aged 65 or under. It usually involves a combination of rifampicin and isoniazid for 3 months, or isoniazid on its own for 6 months. Latent

TB is not always treated if it is thought to be drug resistant. Regular monitoring is required to check the infection does not become active. Treatment of latent TB maybe required for immunocompromised patients.

Antituberculosis drugs

Isoniazid:

Side effects: peripheral neuropathy is a common side effect and if this occurs pyridoxine (vitamin B6) should be given.

Rifampicin:

Side effects: liver function disturbance. Rifampicin induces hepatic liver enzymes which accelerated the metabolism of several drugs.

Rifabutin is a newly introduced rifamycin and is indicated for prophylaxis against *M. avium* complex in patients with a low CD4 count. It is also used for the treatment of non-tuberculous mycobacterial disease and pulmonary TB.

Pyrazinamide:

Side effects: liver toxicity

Ethambutol:

Side effects: visual disturbance including loss of acuity, colour blindness and restriction of visual fields.

Streptomycin:

Side effects: hypersensitivity reactions. Streptomycin is used in cases of resistant organisms.

Monitoring

Isoniazid, Rifampicin and Pyrazinamide are associated with liver toxicity so hepatic function needs to be monitored. Renal function should be checked before treatment with anti-tuberculous drugs and appropriate drug adjustments made. Streptomycin or Ethambutol should be avoided in patients with renal impairment or the dose should be adjusted and drug concentration monitored.

Multi-drug resistant TB (Vank's disease):

This is a form of TB caused by bacteria that are resistant to treatment with at least two of the first-line antituberculous drugs, isoniazid and rifampicin. It is becoming an increasingly serious worldwide problem. It involves prolonged treatment with second line agents which are often less effective. Second line drugs available for infections caused by resistant organisms, or when first line drugs cause unacceptable side effect include amikacin, capreomycin, cycloserine, newer macrolides, moxifloxacin and protionamide. Multi-drug resistant TB should be treated by a specialist physician.

CHAPTER 6

Antimicrobials – antifungals

John Steele and Jenny Taylor

Key Topics

- Introduction
- Oral fungal infections
- Anti-fungal drug treatment
- Implications for dental practitioners

Learning Objectives

- To be familiar with the potential drug interactions of anti-fungal medications used to treat oral infections.
- To be aware of the risk factors for oral candidosis.

Essential Dental Therapeutics, First Edition. Edited by David Wray.
© 2018 John Wiley & Sons Ltd. Published 2018 by John Wiley & Sons Ltd.
Companion Website: www.wiley.com/go/wray/dental-therapeutics

Introduction

This chapter discusses the therapeutic agents used to treat fungal infections (mycoses) and to consider the implications for the dental practitioner. Initially, a broad overview of the various types of fungal infections will be provided. This will include a section specifically relating to those fungal infections that may present in the oral cavity. Then the different classification of antifungal medications will be summarized.

Fungal infections are more commonly seen in patients who are immunocompromised resulting in an increased susceptibility to acquiring an infection. Patients undergoing chemotherapy as part of cancer treatment or taking immunosuppressant medication (e.g. after an organ transplant or for an autoimmune condition) can become immunocompromised. In addition, patients diagnosed with an immunocompromising disease (e.g. HIV) or diabetes are also at risk of a weakened immune system. Specific local factors can also predispose an individual to oral fungal infections and these will be discussed later. The chapter's key topics are listed in Table 6.1.

Aspergillosis

Aspergillosis is acquired from inhaling the aspergillus mould which is found in vegetation and crops as well as within the home in, for example air conditioning units. It mainly affects the respiratory system but can affect other organs such as the heart and skin in immunocompromised individuals. It can cause infection, growth of the fungus in the lungs or may initiate an allergic response.

Table 6.1 Key topics
Aspergillosis
Blastomycosis
Cryptococcosis
Histoplasmosis
Oral fungal infections
Skin and nail infections
Antifungal drugs
Implications for dental practitioners

There are different forms of the infection including, among others, aspergilloma, invasive aspergillosis, chronic cavitating aspergillosis and chronic fibrosing aspergillosis.

Clinical features

Symptoms include cough, haemoptysis, weight loss and fatigue.

Treatment

Single aspergillomas may be amenable to surgery. The drug treatment of choice for aspergillosis is voriconazole. Amphotericin is an alternative. Refractory infections can be treated with caspofungin, itraconazole or posaconazole.

Blastomycosis

Blastomycosis is caused by the fungus *Blastomyces dermatitidis* which is found in moist soil and decomposing vegetation. The infection is acquired through inhaling fungal spores.

Clinical features

Many people who inhale the spores do not become symptomatic. Those who do develop symptoms generally develop a flu-like illness: fever, cough and muscle and joint pain.

Treatment

The drug treatment of choice is either amphotericin or itraconazole.

Cryptococcosis

Cryptococcal infections are caused by either *Cryptococcus neoformans* or *Cryptococcus gattii* both of which are fungi that are found in soil. They can infect the lungs and nervous system. Cryptococcal meningitis can be life-threatening especially in an immunocompromised patient with HIV infection. Fungal growths (cryptococcomas) can develop within organs.

Clinical features

Respiratory symptoms include a cough, fever and dyspnoea. Neurological symptoms include those seen in meningitis such as headache, photophobia, neck pain, nausea and vomiting.

Treatment

For cryptococcal meningitis or severe pulmonary infections the treatment of choice is intravenous amphotericin in combination with intravenous flucytosine followed by fluconazole. Mild-moderate pulmonary infections can be treated with fluconazole alone. Surgery can sometimes be required to remove fungal growths.

Histoplasmosis

Histoplasmosis is caused by the *Histoplasma* fungus which is found in soil particularly where there are bird or bat droppings. It is acquired through the airborne route and inhaled. Many people who inhale the spores have subclinical infection and do not require treatment. However, histoplasmosis can be a serious infection for the immunocompromised individual.

Clinical features

Many people have no symptoms. Those that are affected often experience a flu-like illness (fever, cough, fatigue, aches) and many do not require treatment as the infection is self-limiting and resolves of its own accord.

Treatment

Those patients that do require treatment may need intravenous amphotericin for severe infections or can be treated with itraconazole if they are immunocompetent and they have a less severe non-meningeal infection.

Oral fungal infections

Overview

In general, oral fungal infections tend to be attributed mainly to the *Candida* genus. *C. albicans* is the most common form that is pathogenic however it should be noted that it exists as a harmless commensal in the mouth in up to 80% of the healthy population. It therefore acts as an opportunistic pathogen. *C. albicans* is also implicated with oesophageal, vulvovaginal and penile candidosis. Other oral *Candida* species include *C. tropicalis, C. glabrata, C. parapsilosis, C. krusei* and *C. dubliniensis* among others.

Risk factors for oral candidosis are summarized in Table 6.2. (This is not an exhaustive list.)

Various forms of oral candidoses can present clinically as intraoral lesions which can appear red or white. These are summarized in the following subsections.

Pseudomembranous candidiasis

This presents as white lesions, which appear as creamy white flecks that can be scraped off often leaving an erythematous base. It is known

Table 6.2 Risk factors for oral candidosis

Local factors	Systemic factors
Dry mouth	Oral broad spectrum antibiotics
Use of topical corticosteroids (including steroid asthma inhalers)	HIV Diabetes mellitus
Removable dental appliances (including dentures)	Haematinic deficiencies Immunosuppressant medications
Smoking	Chemotherapy agents Extremes of age Malnutrition

44 / Essential dental therapeutics

colloquially as thrush. It can be seen in severely immunocompromised patients, in patients who do not rinse their mouth out after using steroid inhalers and in patients treated with systemic broad spectrum antibiotics. Polyene, imidazole or triazole antifungals can be used to treat the infection. Advice regarding rinsing after steroid inhalers should also be given.

Acute/chronic erythematous candidiasis

Denture stomatitis:

This affects the mucosa that is directly in contact with removable dental appliances such as dentures or orthodontic appliances. While the mucosa can appear red and inflamed, it is often asymptomatic. Poor denture hygiene can precipitate this condition.

Median rhomboid glossitis:

This presents as a rhomboid shaped red patch in the midline dorsal surface of the tongue. Current thinking is that it is caused by a candidosis that infiltrates the site of the lesion. Systemic azoles are the medication of choice.

Angular cheilitis:

Inflammation of the angles of the mouth can be attributed to both *Candida* species as well as *Staphylococci* or *Streptococci*. The appearance of this lesion is of cracked, red, fissured and crusted corners of the mouth that can be painful. It is often seen in denture wearers where the occlusal vertical dimension is reduced as well as in those patients with haematinic deficiencies. Topical imidazoles such as miconazole can be used to treat this infection. Miconazole is active against both *Candida* and *Staphylococci* or *Streptococci*. For specific treatment for Staphylococcal infections please see the Antibacterial section.

Chronic hyperplastic candidiasis:

This potentially malignant lesion is sometimes known as candidal leukoplakia. It presents as a persistent white or white/red raised patch which can't be scraped off. It usually develops at the labial commissures but can affect other intra-oral sites. It is thought to be caused by infiltration of *Candida*

Table 6.3 Clinical presentations of Tinea

Tinea subtype	Site affected
Tinea barbae	Beard
Tinea capitis	Scalp and hair
Tinea corporis	Skin excluding scalp, beard, groin, feet and toes
Tinea cruris	Skin of groin and perineum
Tinea pedis	Soles of feet Between toes
Tinea unguium (aka onychomycosis)	Nails of hands or feet
Tinea versicolor (pityriasis versicolor)	Skin

hyphae into the epithelium causing inflammatory and occasionally dysplastic changes. The lesions are usually seen in smokers. The treatment of choice is a systemic triazole such as fluconazole. Because of its malignant potential, lesions should be biopsied to assess for epithelial dysplasia. Initial treatment with a systemic antifungal prior to biopsy could be considered if clinically suspicious since the presence of fungal hyphae in the lesion interferes with the assessment of the dysplasia. If treatment occurs after biopsy investigation that has identified dysplastic changes then a further biopsy should be undertaken to evaluate if there has been resolution/improvement in the grade of dysplasia.

Skin and nail infections

Tinea, which is also known as ringworm, encompasses a number of different presentations as shown in Table 6.3.

A variety of topical and systemic agents can be used in treatment of these conditions. It should be noted that tinea unguium can be particularly difficult to treat and may need a prolonged course of systemic antifungals.

Antifungal drug treatment

There are essentially two ways by which medication can be used to treat a fungal infection. The medication can have either fungistatic or fungicidal activity.

Fungistatic activity: inhibits and prevents further growth of a fungus without destroying it. Fungicidal activity: kills/destroys fungi organisms.

Fungi exist as either filamentous moulds comprising hyphae or as yeasts that reproduce by budding. Antifungal medication acts against fungal cell membranes by binding to and disrupting them (polyenes) or blocking ergosterol formation (azoles). Griseofulvin blocks intracellular microtubules.

There are a number of different classes of antifungal medication and these are discussed in the following subsections.

Triazole antifungals

The triazoles include fluconazole, itraconazole, posaconazole and voriconazole. They are taken orally or by intravenous infusion. They are fungistatic. They are systemically absorbed and secreted in saliva providing effective, continuous antifungal activity between doses.

Side effects:

Side effects of these agents include gastro-intestinal disturbances (nausea, vomiting, abdominal pain, diarrhoea, dyspepsia, flatulence), rash, taste disturbance, hepatic and blood disorders including leucopenia.

Caution is recommended when considering prescribing these medications in patients with hepatic and renal impairment. Itraconazole should be avoided in patients who have a history of heart failure and ventricular dysfunction.

Imidazole antifungals

The imidazoles include drugs such as clotrimazole, econazole, ketoconazole, miconazole and tioconazole and they are fungistatic. They are all topical preparations apart from ketoconazole which can be taken orally.

Side effects:

With ketoconazole and miconazole side effects are similar to the triazole antifungals. It should be noted that there is a very rare risk of potentially life-threatening hepatotoxicity with ketoconazole if the course is given for longer than 10 days. Clotrimazole and econazole are used in the treatment of vaginal candidiasis and can damage latex condoms and diaphragms.

Polyene antifungals

The polyene antifungals include amphotericin and nystatin. They have fungicidal activity. They act by binding to ergosterol in the fungal cell wall and this results in a disruption of the cell membrane structure. In contrast to most azole antifungals, these agents are not systemically absorbed and so oral administration has a purely topical and short-term action. Amphotericin, however, can be administered intravenously.

Side effects:

Side effects of amphotericin include anorexia, nausea and vomiting, diarrhoea, renal toxicity, cardiovascular toxicity and abnormal liver function. There is a lipid formulation of amphotericin available which is less toxic but is more expensive. Nystatin side effects include an unpleasant taste, oral sensitization and irritation and nausea.

Echinocandin antifungals

The echinocandin antifungals include drugs such as anidulafungin, caspofungin and micafungin. They are used in the management of invasive candidiasis. Caspofungin is also used to treat invasive aspergillosis. They are administered by intravenous infusion.

Side effects:

Side effects of these agents include nausea, vomiting, diarrhoea, rash, hepatic dysfunction and blood disorders.

Other antifungals

There are a number of other antifungal drugs such as flucytosine, griseofulvin and terbinafine. Chlorhexidine also has antifungal properties. Terbinafine is both fungistatic and fungicidal and is the first-line systemic agent in the management of tinea unguium and is also used topically in the treatment of ringworm.

Side effects:

The side effects of these agents are very similar to the other classes of antifungal medications potentially causing abdominal symptoms, hepatic toxicity, blood disorders (e.g. thrombocytopaenia, leucopaenia) and rashes. Toxic epidermal necrolysis and erythema multiforme/Stevens-Johnson syndrome have been reported.

Implications for dental practioners

Dental practitioners (dental surgeons and dental care professionals) are ideally placed to identify oral fungal infections which may represent a serious underlying systemic medical condition.

Consideration should be given to interactions with other medications when prescribing antifungals in dental practice. The most commonly prescribed antifungals include nystatin, miconazole and fluconazole. The latter two medications should not be prescribed concomitantly with statins or coumarins (warfarin) as they can lead to myopathy (muscle weakness) and an increased bleeding risk respectively. In particular, fluconazole, itraconazole, voriconazole and miconazole enhance the effect

Table 6.4 Oral side effects of antifungal medications

Side effect	Implicated antifungal medications
Cheilitis	Voriconazole
Dry mouth	Caspofungin, Posaconazole
Gingivitis	Voriconazole
Glossitis	Griseofulvin, Voriconazole
Mouth ulcers	Posaconazole
Oral irritation and sensitization	Nystatin
Taste disturbance	Fluconazole, Itraconazole, Miconazole, Caspofungin, Micafungin, Griseofulvin, Terbinafine

of coumarins – they increase the patient's INR and make them more prone to bleed. Even though miconazole is used topically as a gel or cream in dentistry and is not absorbed in therapeutic quantities, enough is absorbed to interfere with concurrent coumarin therapy and so topical agents containing miconazole should also be avoided.

It is also important to appreciate the potential oral side effects of antifungal medications. Table 6.4 lists some oral side effects and the implicated therapeutic agents.

CHAPTER 7
Antimicrobials – antivirals

John Steele and Jenny Taylor

Key Topics

- Herpesvirus infections
- Human immunodeficiency virus (HIV)
- Implications for dentistry

Learning Objectives

- To be familiar with the drug treatment for herpes simplex infections
- To be aware of the potential oral side effects of highly active anti-retroviral therapy (HAART).

Essential Dental Therapeutics, First Edition. Edited by David Wray.
© 2018 John Wiley & Sons Ltd. Published 2018 by John Wiley & Sons Ltd.
Companion Website: www.wiley.com/go/wray/dental-therapeutics

Introduction

There are many viruses that are pathogenic to the human body. These range from mild self-limiting infections in an immunocompetent individual – for example common cold – to potentially life-threatening/life-changing infections such as HIV, Ebola virus disease (EVD) and Zika virus disease.

This chapter will provide a concise summary of those viral infections that have drug treatment available as shown in Table 7.1 and then implications for dentists/dental care professionals will be discussed.

There are many other viruses that can affect the oral cavity and associated structures including Coxsackie viruses (hand, foot and mouth disease, herpangina), human papilloma virus (HPV), measles and paramyxovirus (mumps). These will not be discussed here as there are no specific therapeutic agents available although imiquimod is sometimes used off-label to treat oral warts. There are vaccines now available to prevent HPV infection but they will not be discussed in this chapter.

Viral infections can cause non-specific systemic symptoms such as malaise and fever. General supportive advice is recommended such as fluids, rest and regular anti-pyrexial therapies (paracetamol or ibuprofen).

Hepatitis (viral)

The most common types of viral hepatitis are hepatitis A, hepatitis B (HBV) and hepatitis C (HCV). There are two others identified namely hepatitis D and hepatitis E.

This group of viruses essentially cause inflammation of the liver and can have other longer-term sequelae such as liver cirrhosis and the development of hepatocellular carcinoma (HBV & HCV).

Table 7.1 Viral infections
Hepatitis (viral)
Human Herpesvirus (HHV) infections
Human Immunodeficieny Virus (HIV)
Influenza
Respiratory syncytial virus (RSV)

HBV and HCV are acquired through contact with infected blood or with bodily fluids (semen and vaginal) through unprotected sex. Antiviral medication is available for HBV and HCV and is discussed below.

Hepatitis B drug treatment

Drugs used in the treatment of HBV include adefovir, entecavir and telbivudine, peginterferon alfa-2a, and tenofovir disoproxil.

For specific Hepatitis B antiviral treatment guidance please see https://www.nice.org.uk/guidance/cg165 from the National Institute for Health and Care Excellence (NICE).

Hepatitis C drug treatment

Anti-viral drugs used in the treatment of HCV include boceprevir, sofosbuvir and telaprevir. NICE has also recently recommended, in draft guidance, newer treatment options including daclatasvir, ledipasvir-sofosbuvir, ombitasvir-paritaprevir-ritonavir with or without dasabuvir (https://www.nice.org.uk/news/press-and-media/nice-recommends-new-treatment-options-for-hepatitis-c).

NICE has paused the guidance for HCV treatment at present so that the newer drugs can be properly evaluated.

Herpesvirus infections

There are eight identified viruses in the human herpesvirus (HHV) group, which are summarized in Table 7.2.

Drug treatment is available for the management of HSV1, HSV2 and VZV infections.

Clinical Features – Oral

HSV1 and HSV2 can cause a variety of clinical appearances. Primary infection is usually a minor self-limiting illness however some patients develop more severe symptoms such as primary herpetic gingivostomatitis. Once acquired, the virus remains with the patient lifelong and can be reactivated

Table 7.2 Viruses in the human herpesvirus (HHV) group		
HHV subtype	**Also known as**	**Clinical disease**
HHV-1	Herpes Simplex Virus 1 (HSV1)	Primary herpetic gingivostomatitis Herpes labialis Genital herpes
HHV-2	Herpes Simplex Virus 2 (HSV2)	Genital/oral herpes
HHV-3	Varicella-Zoster Virus (VZV)	Chicken pox Shingles
HHV-4	Epstein-Barr Virus	Infectious mononucleosis Hairy leukoplakia Nasopharyngeal carcinoma Burkitt's lymphoma Lymphoproliferative disease
HHV-5	Cytomegalovirus (CMV)	CMV infection
HHV-6		Roseola infantum ('sixth disease') Pityriasis rosea
HHV-7		Pityriasis rosea
HHV-8	Kaposi's Sarcoma Herpes Virus (KSHV)	Kaposi's sarcoma

during periods when the immune system is weakened. Recurrence of the virus most often presents initially with a prodromal symptom such as tingling and is then followed by the development of a vesicular lesion usually on the vermillion border of the lips.

HSV has been implicated in triggering an immune mediated response seen in erythema multiforme and for recurrent cases, prophylactic systemic aciclovir should be considered.

HSV has also been implicated in the aetiology of Bell's palsy and systemic antiviral medication can be considered early in the presentation.

Herpetic whitlow describes the appearance of HSV1 or HSV2 when it affects the fingers and was a particular risk to dentists/dental care practitioners prior to the routine use of barrier protection such as disposable gloves. Herpes simplex keratitis can affect the eyes and so eye protection should be worn especially if an aerosol is created when using high speed rotary handpieces.

VZV primary infection is commonly known as chicken pox. Reactivation of the virus is known as shingles and is often a unilateral painful dermatomal vesicular rash. Oral ulcers are also a feature of both primary and secondary VZV. Chronic pain can persist (post-herpetic neuralgia) after the rash from shingles has resolved but the management is beyond the scope of this chapter.

Cytomegalovirus (CMV) infection has symptoms similar to glandular fever or the influenza infection whereby a fever, sore throat and lymphadenopathy are commonplace. Once acquired, it can lie dormant until reactivated due to immunosuppression.

Herpes simplex infections – drug treatment

Aciclovir is a nucleoside analogue drug and is the most commonly prescribed medication for oral herpes infections. It is available in both topical and systemic forms (tablet and intravenous infusion).

It is important to note that the medication should be used in the first few days of the infective episode otherwise it is less likely to be effective.

The usual oral dose for treating primary herpetic gingivostomatitis in a patient over 2 years old is

200mg five times daily for 5 days. The usual oral dose for treating shingles in a patient 12 years and older is 800mg five times daily for 7 days.

Prophylactic dosage regimes are also available for the prevention of recurrent herpes infections and these include aciclovor 400mg BD.

Alternative drugs for treating herpesvirus infections include famciclovir, inosine pranobex, penciclovir and valaciclovir.

Cytomegalovirus infection – drug treatment:

There are various antiviral drugs available to treat CMV infection and include cidofovir, ganciclovir, foscarnet sodium and valganciclovir.

Reported side effects relevant to the oral cavity include taste disturbance (ganciclovir and valganciclovir).

Human Immunodeficiency Virus (HIV)

HIV is a retrovirus that is transmitted through blood or through bodily fluids following unprotected sexual contact. It affects CD4 (cluster of differentiation) cells, which are found on T-helper cells among others. The virus renders the individual immunodeficient and susceptible to opportunistic infections. AIDS (Acquired Immunodefiency Syndrome) is the end stage of the infection whereby the CD4 count has fallen to a critical level.

The types of infections seen in HIV/AIDS are beyond the scope of this chapter and will not be discussed here. It is important to know that all types of infections: bacterial, fungal and viral as well as more exotic infections, can present opportunistically due to the degree of host immunosuppression. They can be much more difficult to treat and can in some cases be fatal due to the extent of the immunodeficiency.

A patient's response to HIV treatment is assessed by monitoring their CD4 count and viral load.

HIV – drug treatment

The mainstay of HIV treatment is using a combination of medications known as HAART – highly active anti-retroviral therapy, that suppresses the replication of and therefore the amount of virus detectable within the body. The aim of treatment is to decrease both the morbidity and mortality rates for HIV infected individuals.

There are various classes of medication used in combination and these are briefly discussed in turn in the following subsections.

Nucleoside reverse transcriptase inhibitors (NRTIs):

These drugs inhibit the replication of the HIV by interrupting the reverse transcriptase process. Examples include: abacavir, didanosine, emtricitabine, lamivudine, stavudine, tenofovir disoproxil, and zidovudine.

Potential side effects include gastrointestinal disturbance (nausea, vomiting, abdominal pain, diarrhoea), pancreatitis, hepatic impairment, life-threatening lactic acidosis and blood disorders including anaemia. Mouth ulceration has been listed as a side effect of abacavir; taste disturbance and pigmentation of the oral mucosa may occur with zidovudine.

Non-nucleoside reverse transcriptase inhibitors (NNRTIs):

NNRTIs also inhibit the reverse transcriptase process but act at a different site on the reverse transcriptase enzyme and so do not compete with NRTIs. Examples of NNRTIs include efavirenz, etravirine, nevirapine and rilpivirine.

General potential side effects of NNRTIs include rash (includes Stevens-Johnson syndrome and toxic epidermal necrolysis), gastro-intestinal disturbance, hepatitis and hyperlipidaemia. Etravirine and rilpivirine may cause dry mouth.

Protease inhibitors:

Protease inhibitors block activation of the HIV protease enzyme, which cuts up proteins to synthesize new HIV particles and therefore prevents the production of new viruses. Examples of this group of drugs include atazanavir, darunavir, fosamprenavir, indinavir, lopinavir with ritonavir, ritonavir, saquinavir, and tipranavir.

This group of antiretrovirals are used with caution in diabetics as they can cause hyperglycaemia and in haemophiliacs as they may increase the risk of bleeding. Lipodystrophy syndrome is a potential side effect as well as gastro-intestinal disturbance, hepatic dysfunction, pancreatitis, blood disorders and sleep disturbance among others.

Specific potential oral side effects include taste disturbances, dry mouth (atazanavir, darunavir, indinavir, lopinavir with ritonavir, ritonavir and saquinavir), mouth ulcers (atazanavir, ritonavir), stomatitis (darunavir, lopinavir with ritonavir) and perioral paraesthesia (ritonavir).

Other HIV antiretrovirals:

There are a group of other HIV antiretrovirals (dolutegravir, enfuvirtide, maraviroc, raltegravir) that can be used in combination with different antiretroviral drugs. General side effects include gastrointestinal disturbance, hypersensitivity reactions, insomnia and mood disturbance (depression, anxiety). Raltegravir has a number of listed potential oral side-effects including dry mouth, gingivitis, taste disturbance and glossitis.

The medications used to treat HIV have potential interactions with medications that general dental practitioners may prescribe. Maintaining up to date information is essential and the use of a web site such as www.hiv-druginteractions.org should be considered.

Influenza

Influenza is a common airborne virus transmitted by droplet/aerosol spread that has many different virulent strains that show seasonal variation. It is highly contagious and can lead to an epidemic most often during the winter months. There have been a number of pandemics with a high mortality rate. Those individuals most at risk include those that are immunocompromised (e.g. immunosuppressant medication, cancer treatment, immunological deficiencies, diabetes etc), pregnant women and those at the extremes of age. Symptoms include coughs, sneezes, fever, weakness, generalized aches and pains including headaches. The symptoms are self-limiting in most cases but in selected cases anti-viral medication may be required.

Influenza – drug treatment

There are various influenza vaccinations available including Haemophilus influenza type b (Hib) vaccine which is administered as part of the childhood immunization schedule in the UK. There are also seasonal influenza vaccines made available to healthcare workers, the immunocompromized, the elderly and those with specific medical conditions (e.g. COPD, diabetes mellitus).

Examples of drugs used in the prophylaxis and treatment of influenza include amantadine hydrochloride, oseltamivir and zanamivir. NICE, however, do not recommend amantadine for the treatment of influenza.

Potential side effects include gastrointestinal disturbance, rash and risk of developing Stevens-Johnson syndrome. There are no specific oral side effects reported with oseltamivir and zanamivir. Amantadine may cause a dry mouth.

Respiratory syncytial virus (RSV)

Respiratory syncytial virus is highly virulent and is one of the main causes of lower respiratory tract infection (LRTI) in infants and young children although can affect any age group. It is transmitted by droplet spread and commonly presents with cold-like symptoms. Most children become infected with this virus as a child and the effects are mild however babies and children with underlying medical problems may have a more serious infection. In babies less than one year of age, cyanosis, nasal flaring, tachypnoea, dyspnoea and wheezing may also be evident. In serious cases, RSV can result in bronchiolitis and pneumonia.

Respiratory syncytial virus – drug treatment

There are two medications available on prescription to treat respiratory syncytial virus: palivizumab and ribavirin.

Palivizumab is a monoclonal antibody that is administered by injection. It is licensed for the prevention of LRTIs in those children who are at high risk. Common side effects include fever and injection-site reactions. Other side effects include gastro-intestinal upset, wheeze, drowsiness and rash among others.

Ribavirin, which is also used in the treatment of Hepatitis C as mentioned earlier, is administered by inhalation for the treatment of RSV in infants. There are some specific side effects that are noted that could occur with inhaled ribavirin and these include bacterial pneumonia, pneumothorax and possibly a worsening of the patient's breathing problem.

Implications for dentistry

Many viruses are spread through contact with bodily fluids. This is especially relevant to dentists and dental care professionals due to the potential spread via blood and saliva. Aerosol spread can occur when using high speed rotary handpieces. Clinicians should practice appropriate cross-infection measures including the wearing of personal protective equipment – for example gloves, masks and visors.

Healthcare professionals should be vaccinated against Hepatitis B according to local guidelines.

Herpetic whitlow can be prevented from being contracted through the use of barrier hand protection in the form of disposable gloves.

Herpes simplex keratitis can be avoided by wearing appropriate eye protection.

Clinicians who undertake Exposure Prone Procedures (EPP) should become familiar with the local needlestick policy to ensure effective aftercare and management including the initiation of post exposure prophylaxis (PEP) in a timely manner.

The side effects of relevance to the oral cavity in relation to HAART include pigmentation, dry mouth, mouth ulceration, stomatitis (including gingivitis, glossitis), taste disturbance and perioral paraesthesia.

CHAPTER 8

Therapeutics of pain management

Roddy McMillan

Key Topics

- Pathophysiology of pain
- Pain management medications
    - Local anaesthesia
    - General anaesthesia and sedation
    - Analgesics
    - Chronic pain medications

Learning Objectives

- To be able to identify the key neurological components of the pain pathway
- To be able to identify the mechanism of action of local anaesthesia
- To be able to identify the key medications used in general anaesthesia and sedation
- To be able to list the key analgesics
- To be able to list the main adjuvant chronic pain medications

Essential Dental Therapeutics, First Edition. Edited by David Wray.
© 2018 John Wiley & Sons Ltd. Published 2018 by John Wiley & Sons Ltd.
Companion Website: www.wiley.com/go/wray/dental-therapeutics

Introduction

In answer to the question, 'what is pain?' probably the most widely used definition is that provided by the International Association for the Study of Pain (IASP), which describes pain as, 'an unpleasant sensory and emotional experience associated with actual or potential tissue damage, or described in terms of such damage'.

In terms of a modern understanding the nature of pain and how it is experienced, in 1968 Ronald Melzack and Kenneth Casey described the '3 dimensions of pain' – in so far as pain comprises three interactive domains: 'sensory-discriminative' (intensity, character, location, and duration of the pain); 'affective-motivational' (unpleasantness and urge to escape the unpleasantness of the pain) and 'cognitive-evaluative' (interplay of cognitions such as prior experiences, appraisal, cultural values and distraction). This was an important watershed in the understanding of pain, as it suggested that the intensity (sensory-discriminative) and unpleasantness (affective-motivational) aspects of pain were not just determined by the magnitude of the painful stimulus, but were also influenced by an individual's intrinsic cognitive functions.

The experience of pain is very subjective and is influenced by many factors such as gender, mood, cultural beliefs, distraction, catastrophizing (negative thinking about the pain experience), and genetics. The physiological processing of pain is a complex interaction between the central and peripheral nervous systems (Figure 8.1)

Nociceptors

The nociceptors are the sensory receptors that detect noxious stimuli, converting these into electrical impulses which are conducted into the central nervous system (CNS) via the Aδ and C fibres. These primary afferent (conducting towards the CNS) Aδ and C fibres are distributed throughout the body (skin, viscera, muscles, joints, meninges), and can be triggered by mechanical, thermal or chemical stimuli. Inflammatory mediators such as prostaglandins, bradykinin, cytokines and serotonin are released from damaged tissues and can directly stimulate nociceptors. Moreover, such mediators can sensitize tissues by reducing the threshold at which nociceptors are activated (the amount of stimulation required to produce a pain signal is reduced) – a process known as 'primary sensitization'.

Dorsal horn of the spinal cord

The Aδ and C primary afferent neurones synapse with secondary afferent neurones in the dorsal horn of the spinal cord. The Aδ and C terminals release a number of excitatory neurotransmitters including substance P and glutamate. Secondary afferent neurones then transmit the signals to the brainstem and brain via the spinothalamic and spinoreticular tracts. The third-order afferent neurones located within the thalamus transmit the pain signals to the higher centres of the brain within the cortex.

In addition to afferent pain signals travelling to the higher pain centres in the brain, inhibitory pain modulation arises in certain areas of the brain (e.g. periaqueductal grey matter), which are highly concentrated with opioid receptors (one reason why opioid drugs are effective analgesics). These inhibitory centres project down to the dorsal horn and inhibit pain signals – the pathways being monoaminergic, with noradrenaline and serotonin acting as neurotransmitters.

While the somatosensory cortex plays an important role in the localization of pain, functional magnetic resonance imaging has identified up to 11 areas of the brain that are thought to be involved in the acute pain experience. This collective is commonly known as the 'pain matrix', and includes the somatosensory cortex, insula, anterior cingulate cortex and thalamus.

Acute and chronic pain

There is debate about when a painful condition is deemed to be acute or chronic. Classically, the arbitrary cut off for acute pain was 3 months duration; however, some suggest that chronic pain can be simply defined as 'pain that extends beyond the expected period of healing'. Within chronic pain conditions, the pain no longer serves its useful protective purpose – acute pain highlights injury or disease, while chronic pain persists, despite the original injury healing.

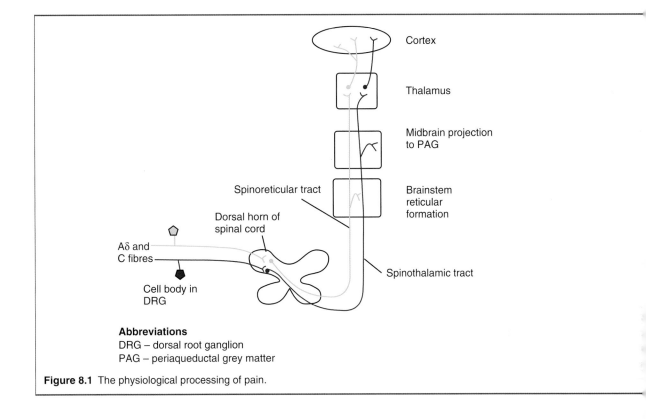

Abbreviations
DRG – dorsal root ganglion
PAG – periaqueductal grey matter

Figure 8.1 The physiological processing of pain.

Neuropathic pains

Neuropathic pains are defined by IASP as, 'pain arising as a direct consequence of a lesion or disease affecting the somatosensory system'. Neuropathic pains are more often chronic in nature and usually present with continuous or persistent pain symptoms; they are often experienced in response to a stimulus that does not usually cause pain (allodynia), or may produce a heightened response to a stimulus that is normally painful (hyperalgesia).

Chronic orofacial pain conditions:

Persistent pains are not uncommon in the mouth and face, and can occur in the absence of any relevant pathology following around 5% of surgical endodontics, or between 3–15% of orthograde root canal treatments. Examples of orofacial pain conditions that are considered to be neuropathic in origin are – burning mouth syndrome (BMS), persistent idiopathic facial pain, trigeminal neuropathic pain and trigeminal neuralgia. Pain-related temporomandibular disorder (TMD) is not thought to be a neuropathic condition and is reported to affect around one-third of the population at some point in their lives.

Role of pain medications within pain management

The World Health Organization (WHO) has promulgated the 'analgesic ladder' as guidance for pain prescribing (Figure 8.2). Initially the ladder was devised for cancer-related analgesia but has since been adopted for all types of pain. The general principle is to start with simple analgesics and depending on response escalate to stronger treatments. When looking at the analgesic ladder, 'non-opioid' analgesics would be medications such as paracetamol and ibuprofen; 'opioid for mild to moderate pain' would be the likes of codeine; 'opioids for moderate to severe pain' would be treatments such as

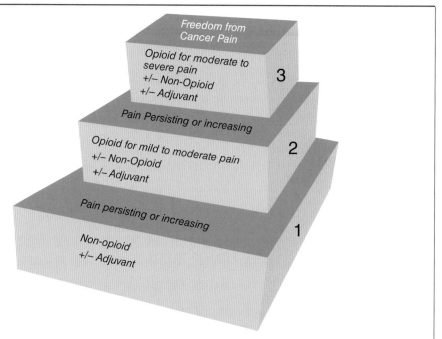

Figure 8.2 The WHO pain relief ladder. *Source:* Taken from http://www.who.int/cancer/palliative/painladder/en/

morphine and diamorphine; 'adjuvant' treatments relates to medications such as amitriptyline and gabapentin. When applying the WHO analgesic ladder to oral and facial pain prescribing, opioids are rarely indicated outside the management of acute pain (e.g. post-operative pain control) or palliative care (e.g. terminal cancer). Prescribing opioids for chronic facial pain conditions (e.g. TMD or BMS) is not recommended – they have limited if any evidence to support efficacy and if prescribed for long courses can cause significant issues with dependency and side-effects.

It is important to remember that it may not be possible to provide any treatments that will completely remove all chronic pain symptoms; rather the emphasis should be more upon pain management. Medications only form one part of chronic pain management – which also includes areas such as: patient education, physical exercises/relaxation techniques, physiotherapy and clinical psychology. The overall aim for chronic pain management is to promote self-management of the patient's condition, and to improve quality of life in spite of the pain continuing to be present.

Local anaesthesia

Local anaesthetics are membrane stabilizing agents; which act mainly by inhibiting sodium influx through the sodium channels in the neuronal-cell membranes. The inhibition of sodium influx results in the nerve action potential not occurring, and signal conduction being prevented (Figure 8.3). Local anaesthetic agents bind more readily to sodium channels in activated, excitable membranes, such as those associated with the nociceptive fibres.

Local anaesthetic agents are split into 'amide' and 'ester' types – determined by their molecular structure. The majority of local anaesthetics currently used in dentistry are amide-type agents (e.g. lidocaine, articaine, prilocaine) compared to a relative few ester-type drugs (e.g. procaine, benzocaine, cocaine) – due in part to an increased level of allergic reactions noted in the older ester-type agents.

Local anaesthetics are weakly alkaline bases which usually exist as hydrochloride salts, thus allowing them to exist in an aqueous solution. Therefore, local anaesthetics are either in a protonated (ionized), or unprotonated (unionized)

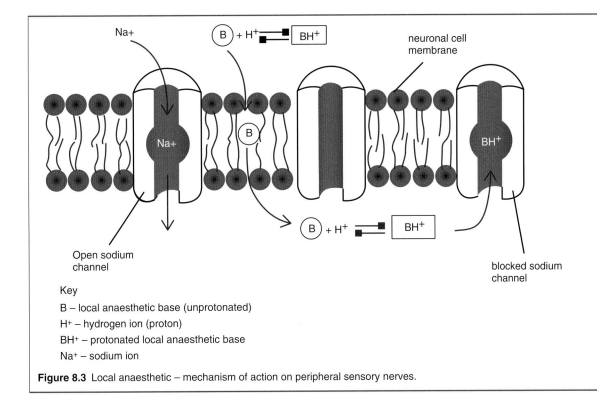

Key

B – local anaesthetic base (unprotonated)

H+ – hydrogen ion (proton)

BH+ – protonated local anaesthetic base

Na+ – sodium ion

Figure 8.3 Local anaesthetic – mechanism of action on peripheral sensory nerves.

form – with only the unprotonated form readily diffusing across cell membranes. Once the unprotonated base enters the cell, it ionizes to the active protonated form, which in turn binds to the sodium channels. The protonated form of the drug does not readily pass through the cell membrane, thus trapping it within the cell (Figure 8.3).

Acidotic tissues, such as those associated with inflammation and infection can partly negate the effect of local anaesthetics – due to the ionization of the local anaesthetic base within the tissues – thus reducing the amount of unionized anaesthetic that can penetrate the nerve-cell membrane.

Although all nerve fibres can be affected by local anaesthetics, on account of differences in nerve diameter and myelination, there are differing sensitivities to local anaesthetic blockade. Type B fibres (sympathetic nerves) are the most sensitive, followed by C fibres (pain), Aδ (temperature), Aγ (proprioception), Aβ (touch and pressure), with the least sensitive being Aα (motor). This 'differential blockade' explains why dental anaesthesia removes

the sensation of pain, but often doesn't prevent the experience of pressure or movement.

Local anaesthetic agents used in dentistry vary in their potencies, and as a result exist in solutions for injection of variable concentration (Table 8.1). Some agents such as lidocaine, dilate vasculature, hence are administered with a vasoconstrictor such as adrenaline, in order to hold the anaesthetic longer in the target tissue and increase effectiveness. On the other hand, anaesthetics such as mepivacaine and bupivacaine don't dilate blood vessels, hence can be administered as effective 'plain' solutions. Some agents are used as a topical anaesthetic – benzydamine hydrochloride is a locally active nonsteroidal anti-inflammatory agent which has local anaesthetic and analgesic properties. Benzydamine comes in a 0.15% solution as an oral rinse or spray, and is used as a palliative agent for a wide range or painful oropharyngeal conditions. Lidocaine can be applied topically to painful oral lesions as either a 5% water-miscible ointment, or as a 10% pump spray.

Table 8.1 Converting concentration to dose

Concentration (%)	Dose (mg/mL)
3	30
2.5	25
2	20
1	10
0.5	5
0.025	2.5
0.0125	1.25

Metabolism and excretion

Ester and amide anaesthetics differ in their pharmacokinetics. Ester-type agents (with the exception of cocaine which is hydrolysed in the liver) are rapidly metabolized by plasma esterases, and consequently have a short half-life. Excretion of ester-type anaesthetics is renal.

Amide-type agents are metabolized by amidases in the liver, a slow process which results in a longer half-life, which can lead to accumulation of the drug and toxicity if repeated boluses or infusions are given.

Adverse effects of local anaesthetics in dentistry

Local anaesthetics are widely and relatively safely used in many aspects of dentistry. Adverse effects associated with the placement of local anaesthetics can be as a result of local trauma following injection, for example haematoma or nerve injury through direct trauma from the needle, or as a result of trauma through chemical action.

Intravascular infiltration of an anaesthetic containing adrenaline (e.g. lidocaine with adrenaline) can result in transient adrenaline associated symptoms, such as tachycardia, sweating and rapid breathing.

Chemical trauma can result from local anaesthetic drugs and can result in demyelination, degeneration and inflammation of the nerve fibres – some studies suggest such chemical injury seems to be more common in the more concentrated solutions (e.g. articaine), compared to less concentrated agents (e.g. lidocaine). Studies show that chemical trauma resulting in persistent anaesthesia or paraesthesia following inferior dental blocks ranges between 1 in 26,762 and 1 in 160,571 cases. Spontaneous recovery is thought to occur in 85% to 94% of such cases.

Although toxic overdose following administration of local anaesthetics in dentistry is very rare, it is important to be aware of the maximum doses of the agents used in dentistry (Table 8.2). Local anaesthetics given in overdose can result in cardiac arrhythmias, central nervous system and respiratory depression; which can be exacerbated by the presence of concomitant opioid therapy, sedatives or hypercapnia.

Although adverse reactions to local anaesthetics are not particularly uncommon, true allergic reactions are very rare. Most true allergies are as a result of hypersensitivity to the metabolic breakdown products of ester-type anaesthetics such as procaine. Therefore, amide-type agents are often used as an alternative in patients who react with the ester anaesthetics.

General anaesthesia

General anaesthesia is the medical induction of a reversible coma, with associated complete analgesia, loss of protective reflexes, loss of muscle tone and amnesia. Medications used to induce general anaesthesia can be either inhalational vapours (e.g. sevoflurane, isoflurane), or solution for injection (e.g. propofol, etomidate). Often anaesthetists will administer a combination of different anaesthetic agents to anaesthetize a patient, for example propofol to induce and sevoflurane to maintain anaesthesia. During the anaesthetic process, additional agents are given to stabilize the patient, such as: oxygen, nitrous oxide, muscle relaxant (e.g. suxamethonium), and sedatives (e.g. midazolam).

Mode of action

The pharmacodynamics of general anaesthetic agents are not as yet fully understood. Most recently, studies suggest that general anaesthetics exert their effect by activation of inhibitory central

Agent	Maximum dose (mg/kg) with adrenaline	Maximum dose (mg/kg) plain (no adrenaline)	Approximate duration of action (minutes)
Lidocaine	7	4	90–200
Articaine	7	N/A	60–230
Prilocaine	9	6	90–240
Bupivacaine	3	2	180–600
Mepivacaine	7	5	120–240
Ropivacaine	3	2	180–600
Procaine	10	7	60–90

Table 8.2 Maximum dosages of local anaesthetics in dentistry/oral surgery

nervous system (CNS) receptors, coupled with activation of the excitatory CNS receptors.

Several anaesthetics (e.g. propofol and sevoflurane) have been found to act upon γ-Aminobutyric acid A (GABA$_A$) receptors. Other target receptor types suggested to play a role in anaesthesia include glycine receptors, potassium and sodium channels.

Metabolism and excretion

Inhalational anaesthetic agents are eliminated via exhalation from the lungs – and as a result recovery is often relatively slow. Intravenous anaesthetic agents such as propofol are metabolized in the liver and are distributed quickly throughout the peripheral tissues, resulting therefore in a short duration of action and rapid recovery.

Sedation

Nitrous oxide

Nitrous oxide is a colourless gaseous compound with the chemical formula N_2O. Nitrous oxide can be used as a carrier gas along with oxygen for more potent general anaesthetic vapours such as sevoflurane or isoflurane (nitrous oxide is not potent enough as a stand-alone general anaesthetic). Nitrous oxide has analgesic properties hence is often used as an inhalational 50% mixture with oxygen – used as an analgesic in situations such as myocardial infarction, trauma and childbirth.

Nitrous oxide is often administered in the practice of dentistry as a sedating and analgesic agent. The process known as 'relative analgesia' is the administration of a titrated inhaled combination of nitrous oxide and oxygen in order to provide conscious sedation in dental patients. Nitrous oxide is generally considered to be a very safe form of sedation, with only mild and transient side effects such as blurred vision, confusion and hypotension.

Benzodiazepines

Midazolam:

Midazolam is a short-acting benzodiazepine solution which can be administered via intravenous, intramuscular, subcutaneous, buccal or nasal routes. In dentistry, midazolam is most commonly used for conscious sedation; however, it can be used for a variety of other purposes such as a premedication, sedative for combined anaesthesia or for the treatment of status epilepticus. Midazolam when administered intravenously begins to work within 5 minutes with a fairly quick recovery relative to other benzodiazepines – effects usually last between 1 to 6 hours.

Midazolam is a GABA$_A$ receptor agonist and thus results in sedation, respiratory depression, hypotension, anxiolysis, anterograde amnesia, muscle relaxation and cessation of epileptic seizures.

Midazolam is metabolized in the liver by the cytochrome P450 enzymes and glucuronide conjugation. The elimination half-life of midazolam is between 1 and 4 hours, with potentially longer elimination in the elderly and children. Overdose of midazolam can be potentially life threatening. Flumazenil is an injectable $GABA_A$ receptor antagonist which competes with benzodiazepines such as midazolam – thus reversing the effects of an overdose.

Diazepam:

Diazepam is a long-acting benzodiazepine which acts as a $GABA_A$ receptor agonist – it can be administered by oral, intravenous, intramuscular or rectal routes. The onset of action is rapid (fairly similar to midazolam); however, the recovery period is much longer – with a half-life of several days with the possibility of 'rebound' sedation. These effects are mainly due to the fact that very little diazepam is excreted unchanged, with most of the drug being metabolized by the liver cytochrome system into several active metabolites, for example desmethyl-diazepam. Due to these pharmacokinetic properties diazepam has limited use in contemporary dentistry.

Temazepam:

Temazepam is an intermediate-acting benzodiazepine which is used for oral sedation in dentistry, insomnia and a surgical premedication. It is the 3-hydroxy analogue of diazepam and one of the active breakdown products of diazepam metabolism. As with other benzodiazepines, temazepam is a $GABA_A$ receptor antagonist which has a similarly rapid onset but is shorter acting than diazepam (half-life between 8 to 20 hours). The drug is metabolized by the cytochrome system and conjugation within the liver prior to excretion.

In the United Kingdom benzodiazepines are categorized as class C controlled drugs; mainly because of their illicit use as recreational drugs. Benzodiazepines are generally only recommended for short-term courses as they carry a high risk of dependency.

Analgesics

The main indications for the use of analgesics in dentistry is for the short-term management of toothache or for postoperative pain control. Paracetamol and non-steroidal anti-inflammatory drugs are the mainstay of such pain control since opioid analgesics do not seem to be particularly effective.

Paracetamol

Paracetamol (acetaminophen) is used as an analgesic for mild to moderate pain in addition to its use as an antipyretic – it primarily is given orally, but can administered per rectal or intravenously.

The pharmacodynamic mechanism of paracetamol is not completely understood, it is proposed that paracetamol inhibits cyclooxygenase (COX), in particular COX-2. This may be the reason why paracetamol doesn't actively reduce the formation of blood clots via thromboxane inhibition. While paracetamol has comparable analgesic and antipyretic qualities compared to nonsteroidal anti-inflammatory drugs (NSAIDs), it has limited peripheral anti-inflammatory effect.

Metabolism is mainly within the liver via glucuronidation, sulfation and hydroxylation and excretion is by the kidneys. The half-life of paracetamol is between 1 and 4 hours, hence the reason for 4 times daily dosing. Paracetamol is very safe with limited side-effects when taking within recommended limits. However, toxicity can occur with excessive intake (in adults a single bolus dose of 10g or 200mg/kg carries a significant risk of toxicity); with toxic by-products of paracetamol metabolism leading to liver damage and potentially death.

Non-steroidal anti-inflammatory drugs (NSAIDs)

Non-steroidal anti-inflammatory drugs (NSAIDs) are a class of medication that is used as analgesics, antipyretics and anti-inflammatories. NSAIDs work as nonselective inhibitors of both the COX-1 and COX-2 enzymes – the majority of NSAIDs providing reversible inhibition with the exception of aspirin which irreversibly inhibits the COX isoenzymes.

Primarily NSAIDs are used as analgesics for mild to moderate pain and as antipyretics, although when used for prolonged periods they are considered to have anti-inflammatory properties.

NSAIDs are generally well tolerated, although they can be associated with a number of potential issues such as: gastroduodenal irritation and ulceration, gastrointestinal bleeds (particularly when prescribed along with warfarin) since they inhibit gastric mucin production, exacerbation of asthma (some asthmatics will have exacerbation of their asthma when taking NSAIDs), allergic reactions and reduced renal perfusion (to be used in caution in renal impairment). With the exception of aspirin which is protective against heart disease, all of the other NSAIDs are reported to slightly increase the risk of ischaemic heart disease when taken over prolonged periods.

Aspirin:

Aspirin (acetylsalicylic acid) is an NSAID that is used as an analgesic for mild to moderate pain, antipyretic and anti-inflammatory. In addition, aspirin has a role as an antithrombotic medication in the management of acute myocardial infarction and prophylaxis against stroke and deep vein thromboses. Aspirin is usually taken orally but can also be provided in a suppository form. Reye's syndrome is a potentially fatal, but rare disease characterized by rapidly progressing encephalopathy and fatty liver. Reye's syndrome can occur following ingestion of aspirin by youngsters – hence aspirin is contraindicated in children under the age of 12 years.

Ibuprofen:

Ibuprofen is an NSAID which is used in the management of mild to moderate pain, pyrexia and inflammation; it usually taken orally, but can be given per rectal or applied topically. Prolonged use of ibuprofen has been associated with an increased risk of gastrointestinal bleeds, stroke and myocardial infarction.

Diclofenac:

Diclofenac is an NSAID used in for mild to moderate pain and as an anti-inflammatory – it is most commonly taken orally, but can be used per rectal, topically or by intramuscular injection / intravenous infusion.

Opioids

Opiates are naturally occurring alkaloid analgesic compounds found in the opium poppy, for example morphine and codeine. Opioids are considered to be medications that possess the same structure and properties as opiates, but are synthetically produced, for example tramadol and diamorphine.

Opiates and opioid medications bind to specific opioid receptors found in the central nervous system and elsewhere. There are three principal classes of opioid receptors, μ, κ, δ (mu, kappa and delta); although as many as 17 other opioid receptors have been identified. The therapeutic effects and side-effects of these medications are determined by their variable affinities to the different opioid receptors.

Due to their euphoriant effects, opiates and opioids can be used illegally as recreational drugs. As a result, many such medications have been listed as controlled drugs – thus putting restrictions on their prescription and storage.

Short-term side-effects of opiates and opioids include drowsiness, respiratory depression, constipation, nausea, vomiting and dry mouth. When used over prolonged periods these medications have associated physical dependency and withdrawal side-effects – reduction and cessation requires being gradual to avoid potentially serious withdrawal symptoms.

Codeine:

Codeine is a naturally occurring opiate (methylated morphine) and is widely used to treat mild to moderate pain. Codeine is often combined synergistically in a compound with paracetamol (co-codamol).

Tramadol:

Tramadol is a synthetic opioid used to treat moderate to severe pain; moreover, it is indicated, as required, for use in breakthrough neuropathic pains. Tramadol exerts its effect by binding to the μ-opioid receptor and inhibiting the reuptake of serotonin and norepinephrine.

Morphine:

Morphine is a naturally occurring opiate that is used for severe pain, including pain associated with myocardial infarction and during labour. It can be taken orally, or via the intramuscular, subcutaneous, intravenous, intrathecal (spinal) or rectal routes. Outside of acute pain management morphine has a limited role in chronic pain management due in large part to dependency issues; it does however form a part of symptom management in palliative care, for example patients with terminal cancer associated with severe pain or distressing shortness of breath.

Morphine is dangerous in overdose and can cause death by respiratory depression. Tolerance to the analgesic effects of morphine occurs rapidly; hence the reason why patients on long-term morphine therapy require a gradual increase in dosage over time to achieve therapeutic benefit.

Diamorphine:

Diamorphine (heroin) is a synthetic opioid analgesic used for severe pain – administered via oral, intranasal, subcutaneous, intramuscular, intrathecal or intravenous routes. As with morphine, heroin also has significant issues associated with overdose, tolerance and dependence.

Chronic pain medications

There is variation between the medications used to manage acute and chronic pains. Analgesics are widely used to manage chronic pains; however, their role is less pronounced when compared to acute pain management – for reasons such as reduced effectiveness of analgesics in many chronic pain conditions, concerns over dependency and side-effects when prescribing analgesics for long durations. Chronic pain management often employs the 'adjuvant' treatments as described by the WHO 'analgesic ladder' (Figure 8.2). These are medications that did not originate as analgesics, but which can have analgesic properties. The most common classes of adjuvant pain management medications are antidepressants and anticonvulsants.

Amitriptyline and Nortriptyline:

Amitriptyline is a tricyclic antidepressant which was originally marketed in the 1960s for the treatment of depression and anxiety; however, it is less commonly used for depression and anxiety now and now has a very prominent role in pain management, for example migraines, fibromyalgia and neuropathic pains.

Amitriptyline is known to interact with 24 different receptor types within the CNS, which include serotonin, noradrenaline, dopamine and muscarinic receptors and transporters. It is considered to be a serotonin-noradrenaline reuptake inhibitor (SNRI) due to its significant predilection for these receptor types.

Amitriptyline is taken orally and is metabolized mainly by the liver to the active metabolite nortriptyline – a drug in its own right, which interacts with 18 of the same receptors that amitriptyline is involved with. Due to their potential cardiac toxicity, both amitriptyline and nortriptyline are contraindicated following recent myocardial infarct and in patients with cardiac arrhythmias (particularly heart block).

Amitriptyline and nortriptyline are generally well tolerated in the dose ranges used for pain management (up to 75 mg at night), which is less than that historically required to manage depression. Side-effects include: drowsiness (often beneficial for sleep disturbance related to pain), dry mouth, blurry vision and increased appetite. Nortriptyline is thought to be slightly less sedative when compared to amitriptyline.

Duloxetine:

Duloxetine is an SNRI that is used in the management of several conditions which include anxiety, depression, stress urinary incontinence in women and neuropathic pains. Previously its role in pain management was centred on diabetic neuropathic pain; although more recently it has been recommended for the management of other neuropathic pain conditions.

Duloxetine is taken orally and is primarily metabolized by the liver cytochrome system. It should not be issued to patients with liver or kidney impairment. The main side-effects of duloxetine are: nausea, dyspepsia, constipation and weight changes.

Carbamazepine:

Carbamazepine is an oral sodium channel stabilizing anticonvulsant which is used for the management of epilepsy in addition to neuropathic pains. In addition to sodium channels, carbamazepine is also a GABA receptor agonist.

In terms of pain, carbamazepine's primary role is in the management of trigeminal neuralgia – a condition which responds promptly and usually profoundly to carbamazepine. Carbamazepine's role in other neuropathic pain conditions is limited.

Carbamazepine is a liver enzyme inducer and hence may increase clearance of many medications, the most notable from a dental perspective being warfarin. Drugs that are more rapidly metabolized with carbamazepine include warfarin, drugs that have decreased metabolism include erythromycin and calcium channel blockers.

More common side-effects include nausea, dizziness and ataxia. Rarely carbamazepine can induce potentially fatal skin reactions – Stevens-Johnson syndrome and toxic epidermal necrolysis – which are more likely in patients who possess the human leukocytic antigen allele HLA-B*1502 allele. This allele is more common in Asians, particularly those of Han Chinese origin – thus genetic testing in this cohort is advised prior to starting the drug, or one can issue an alternative preparation. Carbemazepine can also cause leukopaenia early in treatment and also liver dysfunction and so blood monitoring is required before and during therapy.

Gabapentin:

Gabapentin is an anticonvulsant medication which is also licensed for the management of neuropathic pain conditions – it is thought to work primarily through its effect on voltage-gated calcium channels. Gabapentin is taken orally and is not significantly metabolized, excretion being through the kidneys. Side-effects include gut upset and dry mouth.

Pregabalin:

Pregabalin is an oral anticonvulsant which is also licensed for the management of generalized anxiety disorder and neuropathic pain conditions – working through its effect on voltage-gated calcium channels. Pregabalin could be considered to be similar, although more potent than the older gabapentin. Pregabalin, like gabapentin, is minimally metabolized and is excreted by the kidneys. Side-effects include dry mouth, gut upset and nausea.

Reference

Melzack, R. and Casey, K.L. 1968. Sensory, motivational, and central control determinants: a new conceptual model. In D. Kenshalo, ed., *International Symposium on the Skin Senses*, 423–435. Springfield: C.C. Thomas.

CHAPTER 9

Corticosteroids

Jenny Taylor and John Steele

Key Topics

- Introduction
- Topical corticosteroids
- Systemic corticosteroids
- Implications for dental practice

Learning Objectives

- To be familiar with the use of topical steroids in maintaining oral health
- To be aware of the potential adverse effects of corticosteroids and how they may affect the role of the dentist.

Essential Dental Therapeutics, First Edition. Edited by David Wray.
© 2018 John Wiley & Sons Ltd. Published 2018 by John Wiley & Sons Ltd.
Companion Website: www.wiley.com/go/wray/dental-therapeutics

Introduction

Corticosteroid medications are synthetic agents used either systemically (oral or parenteral route) or topically. They are used to treat inflammation and allergy as well as being used for their immunosuppressive properties.

Examples of conditions requiring steroid treatment include asthma, cerebral oedema, anaphylaxis, inflammatory bowel disease, pemphigus and as part of chemotherapy regimens among many others.

This chapter summarizes the use of topical corticosteroids including those that are licensed for use in and around the oral cavity, systemic corticosteroids and their side effects and the implications for dental practice in terms of steroid cover.

Topical corticosteroids

There are a number of topical corticosteroid preparations available in various different forms including creams, ointments, nasal sprays and eye drops. They act locally to suppress the inflammatory response. They are classified according to the potency of the steroid and the range includes mild, moderate, potent and very potent preparations. Examples include hydrocortisone 0.1% (mild) at one end of the spectrum through to clobetasol (very potent) at the other end. To minimize potential side-effects, the least potent efficacious preparation should be considered.

Compound preparations are also available whereby a corticosteroid is combined with an antimicrobial agent.

Uses in dentistry

Topical corticosteroids have many uses in dentistry from treating oral mucosal ulcerative lesions through to the use of compound preparations to manage, for example angular cheilitis and pulp capping.

Oral mucosal lesions can include oral ulcers (aphthae), lichen planus and mucous membrane pemphigoid among others. Hydrocortisone muco-adhesive buccal tablets can be applied directly to the lesion. Betamethasone 500 microgram tablets can be dissolved in water to make a mouthwash and can be used up to four times daily when lesions are present. The patient must be instructed not to swallow the preparation.

Ledermix® is a dental cement that is a compound preparation containing both an antibiotic and triamcinolone. It can be used to treat reversible pulpitis or for deep caries close to the pulp for both direct and indirect pulp capping.

A compound preparation of miconazole nitrate 2% with hydrocortisone 1% (Daktacort™) can be used to treat angular cheilitis. This preparation may be selected instead of an antimicrobial on its own if there is a significant amount of inflammation at the angle of the mouth.

The off-label use of licensed medications may be considered by a specialist to manage recalcitrant conditions not managed by conventional means. Oral Medicine specialists may consider the off-label use of potent/very potent ointments/creams or corticosteroid inhalers/nasal sprays for example for ulcerative lip lichen planus when systemic immunosuppressants may be contra-indicated or recurrent aphthous stomatitis (recurrent mouth ulcers) respectively.

An intralesional triamcinolone injection, although not technically a topical or systemic use of a corticosteroid, can be used to manage lip/facial swelling in orofacial granulomatosis (OFG). Intralesional injections may also be considered for recalcitrant ulceration.

Topical corticosteroid side effects

Prolonged use of topical corticosteroids can result in thinning of skin/mucosa, depigmentation (may be reversible) and both irreversible striae and telangiectasia formation. They should not be used for untreated bacterial, viral or fungal infections as they can spread and exacerbate the infection. Prolonged use of a potent/very potent preparation may rarely lead to adrenal suppression through systemic absorption.

Topical corticosteroids used to treat oral lesions and corticosteroid inhalers for respiratory conditions may predispose to an oral candidiasis developing. For the latter, patients should be advised to rinse their mouth out with water following use of the treatment.

Systemic corticosteroids

Oral conditions requiring steroid therapy should initially be treated via a topical approach and systemic therapy should not be considered until all topical routes have been exhausted.

The use of systemic corticosteroids in dentistry should be limited to conditions managed by specialists in the hospital setting. Conditions that may warrant treatment with systemic corticosteroids include immunobullous diseases such as pemphigus vulgaris or mucous membrane pemphigoid. Other severe mucosal disease such as major aphthous ulceration or severe erosive lichen planus may also require systemic corticosteroid treatment.

Patients on long-term systemic corticosteroid therapy should carry a steroid treatment card which includes details on diagnosis, dose, prescriber's details and duration of treatment.

Prednisolone

The main types of systemic corticosteroid drugs are: betamethasone, deflazacort, dexamethasone, hydrocortisone, methylprednisolone, prednisolone, prednisone and triamcinolone.

Prednisolone is the most commonly prescribed corticosteroid for treatment of oral and perioral conditions. The equivalent dosages of other corticosteroids are given in Table 9.1

Side effects:

There are an extensive number of potential side effects associated with the use of systemic corticosteroids and a full list is available in the BNF. These include common side effects such as headache, increased appetite, weight gain, mood changes and sleeping problems.

Table 9.1 Equivalent anti-inflammatory doses of different oral corticosteroids*

Prednisolone 5 mg is equivalent to
Betamethasone 750 mcg
Cortisone acetate 25 mg
Deflazacort 6 mg
Dexamethasone 750 mcg
Hydrocortisone 20 mg
Methylprednisolone 4 mg
Triamcinolone 4 mg

*This table takes no account of mineralocorticoid effects, nor does it take account of variations in duration of action
Source: Data from Joint Formulary Committee, 2016.

Table 9.2 Potential side effects of corticosteroids

Glucocorticoid	Mineralocorticoid
Psychiatric reactions	Potassium loss
Diabetes	Calcium loss
Proximal myopathy	Water retention
Avascular necrosis femoral head	Sodium retention
Osteoporosis	Hypertension
Peptic ulceration/perforation	

The side effects can generally be divided into mineralocorticoid and glucocorticoid effects (see Table 9.2) and patients should be treated using the lowest possible dose for the shortest possible time to achieve acceptable efficacy. The effects of steroids are also considered in Chapter 14.

Patients on corticosteroids may require prophylactic treatments to prevent long-term complications. These can include bisphosphonate therapy to prevent osteoporosis and treatment with proton pump inhibitors to prevent gastric ulceration. Further detailed information on the management of patients on corticosteroids is available as a NICE guideline.

Table 9.3 Procedures requiring steroid cover		
Procedure	**Local (LA)or general (GA) anaesthetic**	**Steroid cover required**
General dentistry	LA	No
General dentistry	GA	Possibly (see local guidelines)
Minor dental surgical procedure	LA	No (If on less than 7.5 mg prednisolone daily) Possibly (if on more than 7.5 mg prednisolone daily – suggest double usual dose of steroid on day of procedure)
Surgical procedures	GA	Yes (protocols vary according to severity of the surgery and the dose of daily steroid)

Steroid cover:

Long term (greater than 3 weeks) treatment with systemic steroids can cause reduction in the endogenous production of steroids which may lead to adrenal atrophy and in turn to a reduced adrenocortical response. Dentists should be aware of this problem when planning treatment. While there are no definitive guidelines available, it is accepted that dentists should be aware of the potential requirement of steroid cover for patients undergoing minor surgical procedures with local anaesthetic. A review published in 2004 in the *British Dental Journal* (Gibson et al.) made the suggestions contained in Table 9.3.

CHAPTER 10

Fluoride and toothpaste

Sabine Jurge

Key Topics

- Overview of fluoride, its sources, metabolism and toxicity and its role in caries prevention
- Different fluoride preparations and their use in dentistry
- Different types of toothpastes

Learning Objectives

- To be able to list different fluoride preparations
- To be able to describe safe and effective use of fluoride containing products
- To be familiar with different types of toothpastes

Essential Dental Therapeutics, First Edition. Edited by David Wray.
© 2018 John Wiley & Sons Ltd. Published 2018 by John Wiley & Sons Ltd.
Companion Website: www.wiley.com/go/wray/dental-therapeutics

Introduction

Fluoride is a trace element that is of particular interest to dentists due to its role in the prevention of caries. Fluoride is present in most foods, including drinking water, however the content of fluoride varies significantly. About 90% of ingested fluoride gets absorbed in the stomach and small intestine. It reaches the peak concentration in blood in 20–60 minutes. In plasma fluoride binds to protein and this is not regulated by the body. Adults retain less fluoride than growing children and the excess is excreted via kidneys. The majority, 99%, of fluoride concentrates in mineralized tissues and only 1% is found in the soft tissues. Fluoride can be passed via the placenta and can be found at low concentrations in breast milk.

The role of fluoride in caries prevention became clear in the last century when an inverse relationship between fluorosis and caries intensity was observed in US cities with different fluoride concentration in the drinking water. However, over the past decades it has become clear that the most anti-caries effect of fluoride is from topical rather than systemic use.

Fluoride prevents demineralization of enamel and plays a role in remineralization by forming fluorhydroxyapatite, which is more resistant to an acidic environment. Fluoride ions also directly affect cariogenic bacteria by inhibiting cellular enzymes.

High systemic intake of fluoride in the first six years of the life when the permanent dentition is developing can lead to fluorosis, a developmental disturbance of developing enamel. Enamel becomes more porous and looks opaque, clinically presenting as white horizontal lines or even white or light brown spots on the crowns of the teeth.

Excessive doses of fluoride are toxic and can lead to stomach pain, vomiting, diarrhoea, shallow breathing, weakness, weak pulse, clammy skin, dilated pupils, cyanosis, muscle paralysis and spasms. It causes hypocalcaemia and hyperkalaemia and can lead to death within 2 to 4 hours. From the literature, the probable toxic dose, that can trigger life threatening symptoms and signs and require immediate hospitalization, is 5 mg/kg. In practice, it means a 20 kg child can get seriously ill after ingesting 75 ml of 1000–1450 ppm toothpaste.

Water fluoridation

The fluoride content in drinking water can vary significantly. The optimal fluoride concentration in drinking water that has been found to be most beneficial in reducing dental decay is 0.7–1.2 ppm. If the fluoride concentration exceeds 2 ppm, people are advised to consider an alternative water supply to avoid fluorosis in young children. In the UK about 10% of the population have drinking water with either naturally or artificially achieved optimal fluoride levels.

If the water fluoride concentrations are low in some areas community water fluoridation is practised by adding small amount of fluoride to the water supply. It is considered a safe, efficient and cost-effective way of reducing the caries rate. It works both systemically and topically and is shown to reduce dental decay by up to 29%, however it continues to be a controversial and emotional issue.

Fluoridated milk

Milk fluoridation programmes exist in several countries, but so far there is limited evidence that fluoridated milk has a caries-preventative effect. Fluoride concentration in fluoridated milk varies from 2.5 ppm to 5 ppm. In the UK, there are few schemes where fluoridated milk is available in areas where water is not fluoridated and the caries rate is high.

Fluoridated salt

Fluoridated salt is available in many countries and is especially popular in Germany, France and Switzerland, where 30–80% of available domestic salt contains fluoride. It is recommended by the World Health Organization and is supposed to be cost-effective, however it may not have the desired effect on the target population as children nowadays are recommended to have a low salt intake. On average fluoridated salt contains 225 ppm of fluoride.

Toothpaste

Fluoride toothpastes have been recognized to be the most important way of providing fluoride worldwide. Nowadays most of the toothpastes sold in the United Kingdom contain fluoride. Fluoride compounds used in toothpastes are sodium fluoride, acidulated phosphate fluoride, stannous fluoride, amine fluoride and sodium monofluorophosphate. More recently stannous fluoride sodium hexametaphosphate has been added to toothpastes and are shown to have better coverage and retention to the tooth surface.

Fluoride concentration in standard toothpastes available over the counter varies from 1000 ppm to 1500 ppm, but higher fluoride concentration toothpastes can be prescribed for people with a high caries risk. There is a well-documented dose–response relationship between fluoride concentration and caries-preventive effect. There is approximately 12% caries reduction per every 1000 ppm fluoride concentration in the toothpaste. It means a 2800 ppm toothpaste is 15–20% , and 5000 ppm toothpaste is 30–40% more effective than 1000 ppm toothpaste. The recommended use of different fluoride concentrations in toothpastes is shown in Table 10.1.

Detergents are added to toothpastes to improve cleansing and antibacterial properties. The most commonly used detergent is sodium lauryl sulphate (SLS) for its foaming, cleansing and antimicrobial properties and acceptable taste. It is used in 0.5–2%

concentration. However, occasionally SLS can irritate gingiva and oral mucosa or cause allergy, and therefore less irritant agents can be used, such as steryl etoxylate. These SLS-free toothpastes are proven to be equally effective to the SLS containing toothpastes and can be used as an alternative.

In addition to a caries-preventative effect toothpaste can also improve dentine hypersensitivity. The agents added to toothpaste for this purpose are tubular occludants (strontium chloride and acetate) and nerve desensitizers (potassium chloride, citrate and nitrate). Although strontium- and potassium-containing toothpastes are shown to decrease the symptoms, according to a recent systematic review there is insufficient evidence to tell whether strontium and potassium salts reduce dentine hypersensitivity. More recently calcium sodium phosphosilicate has been researched in desensitizing toothpastes.

Over the recent years whitening toothpastes have become more popular. They contain a higher proportion of abrasives and detergents than the standard toothpastes to be able to remove tougher stains. Often low doses of hydroxyl peroxide or carbamide peroxide are added for their whitening properties and these toothpastes can lighten the tooth colour by one or two shades. Hypersensitivity

Table 10.1 Recommended use of fluoridated toothpastes	
Fluoride concentration	**Recommendations**
<1000 ppm	Not recommended
1000 ppm	Smear of toothpaste for 0–3 years old Pea size toothpaste for 4–6 years old
1350–1500 ppm	Smear or pea size for 0–6 years old with high caries risk Children >7 years and adults (spit out the toothpaste and not rinse)
2800 ppm	>10 years old with active caries Orthodontic appliances Highly cariogenic diet or medications
2800–5000 ppm	>16 years olds with active caries Adults with root caries Orthodontic appliances Overdentures Dry mouth Highly cariogenic diet or medications

Source: Based on *Delivering better oral health: an evidence based toolkit for prevention. 3rd Edition*, Public Health England, 2014.

and gingival irritation occasionally are noted as the side effects.

Fluoridated mouth rinses

Fluoride mouth rinses have been used for many years to prevent dental decay in adolescents and vulnerable adults. Systematic reviews have shown regular use of fluoride-containing mouth rinses can reduce caries in permanent teeth by about 25% compared to placebo ones. It can also benefit patients at risk of root caries.

Typically, a mouth rinse contains sodium fluoride in concentrations of 0.05–0.2% (225–1000 ppm). Also, amine and stannous fluoride formulations are available. Sweeteners and flavouring agents are added to improve the taste. Previously most mouth rinses contained alcohol, however now alcohol-free preparations are more popular. Alcohol stings and if regularly used, may have an adverse effect on the oral mucosa.

Mouth rinses are not recommended for children younger than 6 years due to risk of swallowing and receiving higher than recommended doses of fluoride. A 5 ml teaspoon of average strength over-the-counter fluoride mouth rinse contains about 1 mg of fluoride.

Fluoride gels and foams

Fluoride-containing gels are professionally applied on teeth often with the help of trays. These have been shown to reduce the risk of caries by 28% compared to placebo gels. Acidulated fluoride phosphate gel (AFP) has been the most frequently used fluoride preparation in dental practices until the 2000s, when fluoride varnishes became more popular. AFP gel usually contains 1.23% AFP and has pH of about 3.5. Neutral fluoride gels are also available and usually contain 0.4–2.2% NaF, however the concentrations vary. Recently high fluoride gels (12,500 ppm) have become available for once-weekly self-application at home for certain patient groups.

Fluoride foam is similar to gel, and has the same fluoride concentration and pH. It is applied on the teeth with a tray by dentists or dental hygienists. Compared to gel, foam has an advantage as much smaller quantities are needed for adequate coverage of all tooth surfaces. Studies have shown regular professional use of fluoride foam has caries preventative effect of 24% for primary teeth and 40% for smooth surfaces of permanent teeth, and 75% for white spots around orthodontic braces. There was no preventative effect shown for fissures on occlusal surfaces.

Fluoride varnishes

Topically applied fluoride varnishes have become the most popular operator-applied caries preventative agents used by dental professionals. Fluoride varnishes applied 2–4 times per year can significantly reduce dental caries in both the primary and secondary dentition.

Fluoride varnish contains on average 2.26% sodium fluoride (22,600 ppm). It is well tolerated by young children and can have a prolonged caries preventative effect. Studies have shown fluoride varnish to be more effective than fluoride gels and to reduce dental caries by 74%.

Fluoride tablets

Systemic fluoride intake in the form of tablets, drops, lozenges or chewing gum remains a controversial topic. There have been many studies done, but most of them are of poor quality. They are used in areas with low fluoride content in drinking water. Currently there is limited evidence suggesting fluoride tablets are effective in preventing decay. A recent systematic review suggested fluoride tablets can reduce caries by up to 15% in the permanent dentition. The benefit of fluoride supplements in the primary dentition is unclear. Systemic fluoride intake in children carries a significant risk of fluorosis. A recent randomized controlled study investigating the effects of fluoride tablets on 10–12-year-old children with a high caries risk in Sweden, showed no effect of systemic fluoride intake on caries in an adolescent population. Systemic fluoride supplements for pre-eruptive effect taken by young children possibly carry more risk than benefit and therefore are very rarely used nowadays.

CHAPTER 11

Treatments for dry mouth

Roddy McMillan

Key Topics

- Physiology of saliva in health
- Topical treatments for dry mouth
- Systemic treatments for dry mouth

Learning Objectives

- To be able to list the key constituents of saliva
- To be able to list the main causes of dry mouth symptoms
- To be able to identify the key aspects of dry mouth management:
    - Topical treatments
    - Systemic treatments
    - Preventative treatments

Essential Dental Therapeutics, First Edition. Edited by David Wray.
© 2018 John Wiley & Sons Ltd. Published 2018 by John Wiley & Sons Ltd.
Companion Website: www.wiley.com/go/wray/dental-therapeutics

Introduction

Saliva is of fundamental importance for the maintenance of oral and general health. Essentially saliva consists of water, ions and proteins that are secreted by the salivary glands. In addition to water, saliva also includes: calcium, phosphate, bicarbonate, magnesium, zinc, mucins, enzymes and immunoglobulins. These substances play important roles in oral health and function – lubricating the oral cavity, guarding against infection, protecting teeth from dietary and plaque-related acids, and enabling tasting and food consumption.

Xerostomia is the symptom of having a dry mouth, which can be as a result of reduced or altered salivary flow. In addition, xerostomia can be subjective, when a dry mouth sensation occurs with no clinical evidence of reduced or altered flow. Saliva is produced in large quantities by the major salivary glands in response to food stimulation which aids deglutination. The minor mucous glands produce a smaller quantity of thick mucinous saliva, which coats the mucosa and provides lubrication and comfort. In xerostomia, disruption or loss of this mucous film causes a sense of dryness similar that that which occurs after drinking an acidic fizzy drink regardless of the level of oral moisture. Simple salivary substitution, therefore, does little to restore the oral comfort and this severely limits the usefulness of salivary substitutes or stimulants over simply sipping water.

The prevalence of xerostomia within the general population ranges from 10% to 46%, and appears to be more common in females than males. An objectively dry mouth, with clinical evidence of altered or reduced saliva production, can be as a result of medical treatment or a symptom of an underlying disease. Example causes of xerostomia include: physiological causes (e.g. mouth breathing, anxiety), congenital (e.g. salivary gland agenesis), medical causes (e.g. drug-associated xerostomia, chemotherapy, radiotherapy of head and neck region), or underlying diseases (e.g. diabetes mellitus, Sjögren's syndrome, HIV, Hepatitis C).

Dry mouth can impact negatively on health and quality of life – with the consequences of a chronically dry mouth including: difficulties with eating and speaking, oral soreness, susceptibility to caries and oral candidosis.

Table 11.1 Key points for the management of patients with a dry mouth

Alleviate dry mouth symptoms
Implement measures to reduce the future risk of complications and treat any co-existing conditions (e.g. caries or candidosis)
Improve salivary gland function if possible
Manage any associated systemic disease
Manage patient within a multidisciplinary framework

There should be a systematic approach to the management of patients suffering with a dry mouth. The key points are shown in Table 11.1.

Unfortunately, there is currently a dearth of high-quality evidence relating to the treatment of dry mouth. This is mainly due to a lack of methodologically sound randomized controlled clinical trials, coupled with heterogeneity of the outcome measures and diagnostic classifications used in dry mouth clinical trials.

Topical treatments for dry mouth

The difficulty with topical treatments for dry mouth is that they tend to have low substantivity (products are washed away and swallowed quickly) and do little to restore the integrity of the mucous film, and lack the added benefits held by natural saliva, for example mucins, enzymes and immunoglobulins. The currently available topical dry mouth preparations include rinses, sprays, gels, lozenges and pastilles; the actions of which include: lubrication of the mouth, stimulation of salivary flow and protection of the teeth against demineralization. A summary of currently available topical dry mouth preparations available in the United Kingdom is contained in Table 11.2

Although topical saliva substitutes are considered to be free of side effects, some topical preparations are not deemed suitable for dentate patients as they are acidic (e.g. Glandosane ® spray), and thus potentially harmful to the teeth. Patients who have a discernable difference between stimulated and unstimulated salivary flow rates

Table 11.2 Dry mouth management

Topical Symptom relief	Oral sprays (Trade name/active ingredient/properties) • AS Saliva Orthana® spray – porcine mucin/contains fluoride/neutral pH • Aquoral® spray – oxidized glycerol triesters/no fluoride • BioXtra® spray – lactoperoxidase/no fluoride • Glandosane® spray – carboxymethylcellulose/no fluoride/acidic • Saliveze® spray – carmellose sodium/no fluoride/neutral pH • Xerotin® – carboxymethylcellulose/no fluoride/neutral pH Oral gels (Trade name/active ingredient) • Biotène Oralbalance® - lactoperoxidase gel • BioXtra® - lactoperoxidase gel Pastilles/lozenges (Trade name/active ingredient) • AS Saliva Orthana® - mucin in sorbitol • Salivix® - malic acid • SST® - malic acid Over-the-counter sugar free gums and sweets
Systemic therapy	Pilocarpine hydrochloride tablets (if residual salivary gland function is present) Possibly monoclonal antibody therapies (for Sjögren's syndrome)
Non-pharmacological therapies	Possibly acupuncture Possibly electrostimulation

Preventative therapies	Fluoride supplementation
	
	• Duraphat® rinse - once weekly – 2000 ppm
	• Duraphat® toothpaste
	   ○ 2800 ppm (over 10 years old)
	   ○ 5000 ppm (over 16 years old)
	• Duraphat® varnish 2.26% (22,600 ppm)
	• En-De-Kay® rinse – once daily – 500 ppm
	• FluoriGard® – once daily – 500 ppm
	
	Oral hygiene
	
	• Oral hygiene instruction/hygiene therapy
	• Dietary assessment and advice
	• Denture hygiene advice/management of ill-fitting prostheses

Treatment of oral conditions	Dental treatment to restore carious teeth Antifungal treatment, for example nystatin oral suspension, miconazole oral gel, chlorhexidine gluconate 0.2% oral rinse or fluconazole 50 mg capsules
Treatment of underlying systemic conditions	Liaison with other specialties involved in the patient's care, for example GP, rheumatology, ophthalmology

may derive benefit by stimulating saliva production through the use of a sialogogue, such as sugar-free chewing gum, flavoured pastilles or lozenges. A recent Cochrane review, suggested that there is currently no strong evidence to suggest that any topical treatments are particularly beneficial in relieving the symptoms of dry mouth. The study authors went on to report that there was limited evidence to suggest that oxidized glycerol triester oral sprays may be marginally more efficacious than an aqueous spray. In light of this the choice of topical therapy should be largely based on patient preference.

Systemic treatments for dry mouth

Systemic agents in dry mouth have classically been employed to promote saliva production by means of stimulation of the nerves that supply the salivary glands. The salivary glands are supplied by both the parasympathetic nervous system, which controls salivary flow, and the sympathetic nervous system, which controls the composition. Pilocarpine is a non-selective muscarinic receptor agonist in the parasympathetic nervous system, which acts therapeutically at the muscarinic acetylcholine receptor M3 (stimulates salivation via effect on salivary nerve receptors). The half-life of pilocarpine is 0.76 hours after an oral bolus of 5 mg thus explaining why three times daily dosing is required in order to gain therapeutic benefit. The majority of studies conducted on the use of pilocarpine for dry mouth have been in relation to radiotherapy-induced xerostomia. The optimal dose of pilocarpine in the management of radiotherapy-induced dry mouth was found to be 5 mg orally, three times daily; as higher dosages were found to induce too many adverse effects. Pilocarpine relies on residual salivary gland function in order to provide clinical benefit;

hence the reason why measurement of resting and stimulated salivary flows rates are helpful. The most commonly described side effects of pilocarpine used for dry mouth are sweating, rigours and nausea.

Studies have looked at the use of immunosuppressive drug treatments in Sjögren's syndrome, an autoimmune disease characterized by dry mouth and dry eyes. The biological plausibility of immunosuppressive treatments in Sjögren's syndrome comes from these drugs' abilities to suppress the autoimmune inflammatory process involved in the damage of salivary glands. The immunosuppressive therapies so far assessed in Sjögren's syndrome include: azathioprine, ciclosporin, leflunomide, methotrexate and mycophenolate mofetil. Despite modest benefits being noted with some of the outcomes assessed, there was insufficient supportive evidence to promote the general use of such treatments in Sjögren's syndrome. Currently, there is interest in the use of targeted 'biologic' monoclonal antibody therapies (mAb) in the management of Sjögren's syndrome. The mAb therapies employ antibodies that target specific molecules involved in disease, and stimulate the body's immune system to mount a targeted response against these molecules. Rituximab, a B-cell depleting mAb that targets the CD20 antigen has been studied the most in respect to Sjögren's syndrome. The effectiveness of rituximab in Sjögren's syndrome remains unclear, with conflicting evidence, which may suggest a possible improvement in extra-glandular symptoms such as fatigue, rather than oral dryness.

A summary of the topical and systemic medications for the management of dry mouth is shown in Table 11.2. There is also a summary of other potential remedies and a list of preventive therapies as well as an overview of the management of concurrent conditions. These remedies are also described in detail in other dedicated chapters.

CHAPTER 12

Therapeutics for medical emergencies in dental practice

Roddy McMillan

Key Topics

- 'ABCDE' algorithm
- Medical emergencies of relevance to dentistry
- Medical emergency medication of relevance to dentistry
- The management of medical emergencies in dental practise
    - Adrenal insufficiency
    - Anaphylaxis
    - Asthma
    - Cardiac emergencies
    - Choking & aspiration
    - Epileptic seizures
    - Hypoglycaemia
    - Syncope

Learning Objectives

- To be able to identify the components of the 'ABCDE' algorithm
- To be able to list the medical emergencies of relevance to dentistry
- With regards to medical emergencies in dental practice be able to identify which medications are used, and how they are used for each given condition

Essential Dental Therapeutics, First Edition. Edited by David Wray.
© 2018 John Wiley & Sons Ltd. Published 2018 by John Wiley & Sons Ltd.
Companion Website: www.wiley.com/go/wray/dental-therapeutics

Introduction

Potentially life threatening emergencies in the practise of dentistry are thankfully relatively rare – death in general dental practice is reported only once every 758 practising years. However, non-fatal medical emergencies in general dental practice are far more common, with 1 event every 4.5 practising years. Therefore, it is crucial that dental professionals and their teams are able to identify and manage medical emergencies within their place of work.

The protocols for managing medical emergencies have been internationally agreed by the International Liaison Committee on Resuscitation (ILCOR), European Resuscitation Council (ERC) and the Resuscitation Council (UK). Underpinning the management of medical emergency is the 'ABCDE' approach to assessing any patient who is unwell (Table 12.1).

The underlying principles of managing medical emergencies are shown in Table 12.2.

This chapter looks specifically at the therapeutics of managing medical emergencies in dental practice. The emergencies discussed are shown in Table 12.3.

Choking and syncope don't usually require medication management per se; however, in the interests in completeness they have been included as part of the recognized list of medical emergencies in dental practice.

The medications referred to in this chapter are shown in Table 12.4.

Although not a medication, the automated external defibrillator (AED) is an important part of the medical emergencies kit.

Table 12.1 The 'ABCDE' approach to assessing any patient who is unwell

A – Airway
B – Breathing
C – Circulation
D – Disability
E – Exposure

Table 12.2 The underlying principles of managing medical emergencies

1. Conduct a complete 'ABCDE' assessment and re-assess regularly
2. Treat life-threatening problems before moving to the next part of the assessment
3. Reassess to determine the success of treatment
4. Recognize when to call for help – call for help early
5. Use all members of the clinical team, ideally to be working simultaneously and in a coordinated manner
6. Communicate effectively – use the Situation, Background, Assessment, Recommendation (SBAR) approach
7. The aim of the initial treatment is to keep the patient alive until help arrives

Table 12.3 Medical emergencies in dental practice

Adrenal insufficiency
Anaphylaxis
Asthma
Cardiac emergencies
Choking and aspiration
Epileptic seizures
Hypoglycaemia
Syncope

Table 12.4 Emergency drugs

Adrenaline injection (Epinephrine), adrenaline 1 in 1000, (adrenaline 1 mg/mL as acid tartrate), 1-mL amps
Aspirin dispersible tablets 300 mg
Glucagon injection, glucagon (as hydrochloride), 1-unit vial (with solvent)
Glucose (for administration by mouth)
Glyceryl Trinitrate Spray (GTN), 400 micrograms/dose aerosol sublingual spray
Midazolam oromucosal solution, 5 mg/mL
Oxygen (usually a D size cylinder in dental practice)
Salbutamol aerosol inhalation, salbutamol 100 micrograms/metered inhalation

Emergency drugs

Adrenaline

Adrenaline (epinephrine) is a non-selective catecholamine agonist of all adrenergic receptors. Pertinent to anaphylaxis, adrenaline increases peripheral resistance via $\alpha 1$ receptor vasoconstriction and increases cardiac output through binding to $\beta 1$ receptors. In addition to being a hormone released by the adrenal glands, adrenaline is also synthesized for medical use. Due to adrenaline's potent cardiac effects it is only generally given intramuscularly in cases of anaphylaxis. Adrenaline has a rapid onset and short half-life of around 2 minutes; side-effects include: palpitations, sweating, tremor, anxiety and headache.

Glucagon

Glucagon is a peptide hormone released by the alpha cells of the pancreas – its role is to raise the concentration of glucose in the bloodstream – the effect being the opposite of insulin which lowers blood glucose. Glucose is stored in the liver as the polysaccharide glycogen – glucagon released by the pancreas during periods of hypoglycaemia act to convert liver glycogen stores into glucose, which are released into the bloodstream. As glucagon is unstable in solution, it is stored as a lyophilized (freeze-dried) powder that is reconstituted with water just prior to intramuscular injection.

Once injected it may take 5 to 10 minutes for glucagon to work; moreover, it requires the patient to have adequate stores of glycogen. Therefore, glucagon may be ineffective in some patients, for example anorexics or alcoholics.

Glyceryl Trinitrate

Glyceryl Trinitrate (GTN) is a vasodilating agent commonly used in the management of angina pectoris and myocardial infarction. GTN works by increasing blood concentrations of nitric oxide (endothelium-derived relaxing factor) which in turn leads to vasodilatation – the primary clinical benefit deriving from a reduction in venous return, which reduces the left ventricular workload. The main side effects are related to the potent vasodilation properties – headache, flushing and postural hypotension. GTN can be delivered in a variety of ways – sublingual tablets, spray, transdermal patches or via an intravenous infusion. In the context of medical emergencies in dental practice, sublingual spray is probably the most practical method of administration.

Oxygen

Oxygen should be treated the same as any other prescribed medication. It is used for hypoxic patients to increase blood oxygen saturation and decrease the work of breathing. Oxygen is the most commonly used treatment in medical emergencies and is the most important medication in that context. In general terms, oxygen requires to be carefully titrated dependent on each patient's clinical needs and comorbidities; for example, some patients with hypercapnic (high CO_2) respiratory failure (e.g. chronic obstructive pulmonary disease) require a lower oxygen saturation target of 88–92%. However, in the case of medical emergencies in dental practice all patients who are unwell should initially receive the highest possible oxygen flow – 15 litres per minute through a non-rebreathe mask with reservoir bag. Fine adjustments to oxygen delivery can be made later by the paramedics or the receiving hospital team.

Midazolam

Midazolam oromucosal solution is a short-acting $GABA_A$ receptors benzodiazepine solution which can be administered via the buccal or nasal routes. The first-choice management for status epilepticus is intravenous lorazepam; however, as gaining intravenous access is not considered appropriate in the dental setting, midazolam oromucosal solution is considered the best alternative. Midazolam can result in sedation, respiratory depression, hypotension, anxiolysis, anterograde amnesia and muscle relaxation – many of which will be present in any case during the postictal phase.

Salbutamol

Salbutamol is a quick onset, short-acting β_2 agonist which is most commonly used to treat bronchospasm associated with asthma. Most commonly salbutamol is delivered via an inhaler or nebulizer. Side effects can include: tremor, anxiety, headache, muscle cramps, dry mouth, and palpitations.

Adrenal insufficiency

A patient with adrenal insufficiency may develop profound hypotension due to the stress of a dental treatment or as a result of receiving a general anaesthetic for oral surgery. Patients at risk of developing adrenal insufficiency include patients known to have Addison's disease and patients taking long-term, or who have previously undergone long-term therapy with, systemic corticosteroids.

Patients at risk of developing adrenal insufficiency should be managed in agreement with their medical team as discussed in Chapter 7.

Management

Due to the delay in onset of corticosteroid therapy, the administration of corticosteroids does not play a role in the emergency management of a patient with acute adrenal insufficiency. Instead the role is supportive, while waiting for the paramedics to transfer the patient to hospital for definitive treatment:

- 'ABCDE' assessment
- Lay the patient flat to restore blood pressure/ 'recovery position'
- *Oxygen* – high flow, 15 L via a non-rebreathe mask with reservoir bag
- Transfer patient as an emergency to hospital

Anaphylaxis

Anaphylactic reactions are life-threatening severe type I hypersensitivity reactions driven by IgE mediated histamine release. The symptoms and signs include: flushing, swelling (often lips and face), paraesthesia, itching, wheezing, rapid weak pulse and a profound drop in blood pressure.

Management

- 'ABCDE' assessment
- Lay the patient flat/raise the legs to restore blood pressure
- *Oxygen* - high flow, 15 L via a non-rebreathe mask with reservoir bag
- Intramuscular (IM) *adrenaline* - 1 in 1000/ 1 mg/mL

  - Adult — 500 micrograms IM (0.5 mL)
  - Child more than 12 years — 500 micrograms IM (0.5 mL)
  - Child 6 -12 years — 300 micrograms IM (0.3 mL)
  - Child less than 6 years — 150 micrograms IM (0.15 mL)

- *Salbutamol* 100 micrograms/metered inhalation can be used if patient is wheezing – delivered via a spacer – 10 puffs
- Transfer patient as an emergency to hospital

Corticosteroids and antihistamines are not considered first-line management for anaphylaxis as a result of their delayed therapeutic onset. Due to the high risk of relapse, all patients with anaphylaxis should be sent to hospital by ambulance irrespective of how well they respond to the treatment – in hospital they will receive longer-term management such as corticosteroids and antihistamines.

Asthma

Asthma is a common and potentially life-threatening, long-term chronic inflammatory disease which affects the lungs. The condition is characterized by reversible airflow obstruction and bronchospasm; symptoms include – episodes of coughing, wheezing and shortness of breath. An acute episode of asthma can be precipitated by dental treatment. In cases of patients with 'brittle' asthma receiving dental treatment, it may be prudent to give 2 puffs of prophylactic salbutamol prior to starting their treatment.

Management

- 'ABCDE' assessment
- Position the patient in the most comfortable position for their breathing, for example sitting at 45°
- *Oxygen* – high flow, 15 L via a non-rebreathe mask with reservoir bag
- *Salbutamol* 100 micrograms/metered inhalation delivered via a spacer – 10 puffs
- If patient doesn't respond to the salbutamol – repeat 'back to back' cycles and transfer patient as an emergency to hospital

Cardiac emergencies

Patients attending with cardiac comorbidities in the dental practice are commonplace. The most commonly encountered cardiac problem within a dental practice will be angina pectoris – which presents as central chest pain, which in most cases is due to ischemia of the cardiac muscle through atherosclerotic occlusion of the coronary arteries. Myocardial infarction is the irreversible damage of an area of cardiac muscle, most commonly caused by the disruption of an atherosclerotic plaque in a coronary artery, leading to occlusion of the artery lumen and resultant infarction of the myocardium. Myocardial infarction classically will present with central crushing chest pain (occasionally radiating to the left arm and jaw), pallor, sweating, shortness of breath, vomiting and 'sense of impending doom'. Very rarely patients will present with cardiac arrest in dental practice – most likely as a result of myocardial infarction in patients with known heart disease – presenting as an unconscious patient showing no signs of life.

Management of chest pain in an adult

- 'ABCDE' assessment
- Position the patient in the most comfortable position for their breathing, for example sitting at 45°
- *Oxygen* - high flow, 15 L via a non-rebreathe mask with reservoir bag

- *Glyceryl Trinitrate Spray (GTN)* – 2 × 400 micrograms puffs sublingual
- If myocardial infarction is suspected, or if there isn't a complete response to GTN, then arrange transfer of patient as an emergency to hospital
- If myocardial infarction is suspected – *Aspirin* 300 mg dispersible tablet, sucked or chewed to aid trans-mucosal absorption
- *Repeat GTN* after 5 minutes if no improvement
- If myocardial infarction is suspected, then consider precautionary placement of AED

Management of cardiac arrest in adults

In the case of any patient not showing 'signs of life' (breathing and circulation) – the basic life support algorithm should be employed:

- 'ABCDE' assessment
- Check and open airway
- If no signs of life – call for local help and call paramedics
- Start cardiopulmonary resuscitation (CPR)
  - 30 chest compressions
  - 2 rescue breaths via a pocket mask or bag and valve mask
  - Repeat cycle of 30:2 chest compressions to rescue breaths
  - Attach AED without disrupting chest compressions
  - Continue chest compressions/rescue breaths until – paramedics take over/AED instructs you to stop/too exhausted to carry on and nobody available to relieve you.

Choking and aspiration

Due to the very nature of dental treatment, dental patients are susceptible to choking and aspiration. If a patient has inhaled a foreign body the following signs and symptoms may present:

- Coughing
- Distress
- Short of breath
- Noisy breathing, for example wheeze or stridor

- 'Paradoxical' chest movements/abdominal movements
- Cyanosis

Management of choking and aspiration in adults

- 'ABCDE' assessment
- Encourage coughing
- If possible to safely remove visible foreign bodies from the mouth/pharynx then do so
- If the patient is 'wheezing' then consider use of *salbutamol* as per asthma algorithm
- If they are unable to cough but remain conscious then 5 sharp back blows should be delivered
- If the foreign body is not dislodged following the back blows continue with 5 abdominal thrusts
- If the patient becomes unconscious CPR should be started.

If all of the foreign body material is not removed or accounted for, or the patient remains symptomatic, then they must be transferred as an emergency to hospital. If abdominal thrusts were conducted the patient must be transferred as an emergency to hospital due to the potential for internal injury.

Epileptic seizures

Epilepsy is a group of neurological conditions characterized by epileptic seizures (see Chapter 13). The most common variety of seizure are 'convulsive' (tonic-clonic) characterized by alternating contraction and relaxation of the muscles to produce a jerking/shaking of the body – previously known as 'grand mal' seizures. Tonic-clonic seizures can be caused by epilepsy, although other conditions such as stroke, ethanol intoxication and profound hypoglycaemia can be implicated. Signs and symptoms of a tonic-clonic seizure: include loss of consciousness, drooling, accidental tongue biting, loss of bowel/bladder control, rapid shaking, uncontrollable muscle spasms and temporary cessation of breathing. Most seizures will last only up to a few minutes in duration – with a 'postictal' phase of

sleepiness and confusion being common. Epileptic seizures become a medical emergency when they last longer than 5 minutes in duration, or more than one seizure occurs within a 5-minute period without the person returning to normal between them – a condition known as 'status epilepticus'. Status epilepticus is very serious in so far as it carries a significant mortality – 10% to 30% of patients who experience status epilepticus will die within the following 30-day period.

Management

- 'ABCDE' assessment
- Ensure that the patient is not at risk from injury, but make no attempt to put anything in the mouth or between the teeth, for example airway adjuncts
- *Oxygen* - high flow, 15 L via a non-rebreathe mask with reservoir bag
- Do not attempt to restrain patient's convulsive movements
- After convulsions stop – place the patient in the recovery position and reassess
- If the patient remains unresponsive always check for 'signs of life' and start CPR if no 'signs of life'
- Check blood glucose level to exclude hypoglycaemia
- Indications for sending to hospital are:
  - Status epilepticus.
  - High risk of recurrence.
  - First episode.
  - Difficulty monitoring the individual's condition.
- If status epilepticus (fit lasting longer than 5 minutes or no recovery between fits):
  - Give *midazolam* oromucosal solution (5 mg/mL) via buccal route

▪ Adults	10 mg
▪ Child above 10 years	10 mg
▪ Child 5–10 years	7.5 mg
▪ Child 1–5 years	5 mg

  - Arrange transfer of patient as an emergency to hospital

Hypoglycaemia

Hypoglycaemia is defined as a blood glucose level of <3.0 mmol per litre, although some patients may show symptoms at higher blood sugar levels. Known diabetics should eat normally and take their usual dose of insulin or oral hypoglycaemic before attending for dental treatment.

The signs and symptoms of hypoglycaemia include:

- Shaking
- Sweating
- Headache
- Difficulty in concentration/vagueness
- Slurred speech
- Confusion
- Aggressive/combative
- Unconsciousness
- Fitting/seizures

Children often don't have such obvious features and may simply appear lethargic.

Management

All patients with reduced levels of consciousness should have their capillary blood glucose measured – therefore, a capillary blood glucose meter should be included in all dental emergency kits. In the event where a capillary blood glucose measurement is unobtainable, all known diabetic patients should be assumed to have hypoglycaemia and should be managed accordingly.

- 'ABCDE' assessment (including a capillary blood glucose measurement)
- If patient is cooperative and conscious with an intact gag reflex - give *oral glucose* (sugar (sucrose), milk with added sugar, glucose tablets or gel) - repeated in 10–15 minutes if required
- To prevent relapse after initial recovery consider giving patient complex carbohydrates, for example bread or biscuits
- If patient has reduced consciousness, or is uncooperative or unable to swallow safely – give *buccal glucose gel* and/or *glucagon*

  ○ *Glucagon injection,* glucagon (as hydrochloride), 1-unit vial (with solvent) – reconstitute glucagon with water before injecting intramuscularly

    - 1 mg in adults and children >8 years old or >25 kg
    - 0.5 mg if <8 years old or <25 kg

- If the patient does not respond to treatment, arrange transfer of patient as an emergency to hospital
- start CPR in the absence of 'signs of life'
- Re-check blood glucose after 10 minutes to ensure that it has risen to a level of > 5.0 mmol per litre
- After recovery with Glucagon, patients should be given oral glucose to prevent relapse of the hypoglycaemia

The patient may go home if they have fully recovered and are accompanied – they should not drive. The patient's General Medical Practitioner should be informed of the hypoglycaemic episode.

Syncope

Inadequate cerebral perfusion results in loss of consciousness. Commonly this occurs as a result of hypotension caused by vagal stimulation – also known as vasovagal syncope or a 'simple faint'. These episodes often occur in response to sudden emotional upset or severe pain – not surprisingly such instances are fairly common in the practise of dentistry.

The signs and symptoms of syncope can include:

- Feeling dizzy or light headed
- Weak and slow pulse
- Pallor
- Sweating
- Nausea/vomiting
- Loss of consciousness
- Occasionally patients may undergo a hypoxic fit (self-limiting fitting in response to the transient cerebral hypoxia associated with syncope)

Management

- 'ABCDE' assessment
- Promptly lay the patient flat and raise the legs to increase venous return and improve cerebral perfusion (it is not possible to faint when lying flat)

- *Oxygen* - high flow, 15 L via a non-rebreathe mask with reservoir bag
- If the diagnosis of syncope is accurate the patient should fully recover with the above management within a couple of minutes – if not then reassess using 'ABCDE' assessment and call for assistance

CHAPTER 13

Central nervous system 1 – mood disorders

Alan Nimmo

Key Topics

- Introduction to mood disorders
- Unipolar depression and its clinical management
- Bipolar disorder and its clinical management
- Anxiety disorders and their clinical management

Learning Objectives

- Be familiar with the common signs and symptoms associated with mood disorders
- Be familiar with the common therapies used to manage depression, and the impact they have both on oral health and the safe management of dental patients
- Be familiar with the common therapies used to manage anxiety disorders, and the impact they have both on oral health and the safe management of dental patients
- Be familiar with the issue of anxiety associated with dental therapy

Essential Dental Therapeutics, First Edition. Edited by David Wray.
© 2018 John Wiley & Sons Ltd. Published 2018 by John Wiley & Sons Ltd.
Companion Website: www.wiley.com/go/wray/dental-therapeutics

Introduction

The central nervous system (CNS) is the most complex of all our organ systems, and how it functions is only beginning to be understood. However, drugs that have effects on the central nervous system are some of the most commonly prescribed medications.

There is also a wide range of CNS disorders that may cause oral symptoms or impact on a patient's oral health, oral hygiene and their management in the dental clinic. Also, neurodegenerative disorders, such as Alzheimer's disease, represent a growing concern, particularly with our aging populations, while strokes represent the leading cause of adult disability.

A simple classification of psychological disease is shown in Table 13.1.

Mood disorders are characterized by exaggerated normal responses such as extreme or inappropriate anxiety or obsessive behaviour. In contrast, psychotic disorders are characterized by abnormal and bizarre thought processes. Depression is primarily a mood disorder, but there is a subtype which includes a psychotic component (psychotic depression). Both mood- and psychotic disorders may respond to therapeutic intervention, but personality disorders are not responsive.

This chapter will examine two of the most common CNS disorders, depression and anxiety, the medications used to manage them, and the implications for dental practice. Together, depression and anxiety are referred to as mood, or affective, disorders. It is likely that more than 1 in 4 people will experience one or both of these conditions at some point during their lives.

Depression

Clinical features

Depression is a very common mood disorder, affecting close to 1 in 5 individuals at some point in their lifetime.

All people experience feelings of sadness, loneliness and grief at some points in their lives. These represent natural human emotions in response to life events. In general, people can still function normally while they have these feelings, and they have a sense they will get over these feelings. However, clinical depression, or major depressive disorder, is considered to occur when these feelings persist for longer than normal, are excessive, or are occurring in the absence of any obvious external trigger. Also, depression is a major contributing factor to suicide.

Symptoms may be chronic or episodic. In addition, clinical depression is accompanied by physical, or biological, signs. The defining symptoms are shown in Table 13.2.

Early morning wakening arises due to agitation and anxiety despite persistent tiredness. A lower pain threshold may encourage susceptibility to chronic facial pain.

There are two distinct types of depression: unipolar and bipolar depression. Unipolar depression is the more common form. Here the mood swings are always in the same direction, ranging from a normal mood state to feeling depressed.

The development of unipolar depression can be reactive, occurring in response to some life event or traumatic experience, and chronic stress is considered to be a major risk factor. This type is regarded as a neurosis. However, it may also arise through endogenous events, where no external trigger can be identified. As with bipolar depression, endogenous unipolar depression may exhibit a hereditary tendency. However, approximately 75% of cases of are non-familial, and reflect stressful life events.

With bipolar depression, which affects approximately 2.5% of the population, the mood swings can alternate between feelings of depression and periods of mania. Mania can be associated with a variety of emotions, including irritability, impatience and aggression, and may sometimes include grandiose delusions. It may, therefore, be regarded as having a psychotic component.

A number of factors may impact on oral health. Suffers may neglect routine oral health practices, they may make poor nutritional choices, resorting to 'comfort' foods, and may avoid routine dental care. In addition, drug-induced xerostomia is an issue with many antidepressant medications.

Recently, evidence has emerged of a mechanistic link between oral and systemic disease, and depression. It is recognized that chronic stress represents a major risk factor for depression. This led

Table 13.1 A simple classification of psychological disease

Mood disorders	Psychosis	Personality disorders
Anxiety	Organic (delirium tremens, dementia)	Psychopathy
Depression	Functional (schizophrenia, psychotic depression)	
Obsession		

Table 13.2 The defining symptoms of depression

Emotional symptoms	Biological symptoms
Sadness and apathy	Retardation of thought
Reduced capacity to experience pleasure	Loss of libido
Lowered self-esteem	Sleep disturbance especially early morning wakening
Emotional lability (e.g. anxiety)	Changes in appetite and/or body weight
Reduced motivation	Reduced pain tolerance
Poor concentration and memory	Lowered energy levels

to a hypothesis that the body's response to stress may result in an immune response, and associated release of pro-inflammatory cytokines. It is this pro-inflammatory state that may mediate the behavioural changes. Hence, there is a two-way process: poor oral health, and the associated inflammation, may be a risk factor for depression, while the effective management of depression may improve oral health.

Neurochemical basis of depression

Clinical depression is considered to arise from a neurochemical imbalance in the brain. The broadly accepted theory to explain depression suggests it is associated with a deficiency in the activity of noradrenaline and/or serotonin in the brain.

Drugs that enhance the activity of noradrenaline and/or serotonin, such as tricyclic antidepressants (TCAs) and selective serotonin reuptake inhibitors (SSRIs), will elevate mood and alleviate the symptoms of depression. However, antidepressant drugs will increase the activity of noradrenaline and serotonin almost immediately, but the anti-depressant effects of these drugs may take weeks or months to fully develop. It is considered the anti-depressant

effects of these drugs are associated with adaptive changes within the brain, rather than their direct, pharmacological effects. Deficiencies in serotonin are thought to be primarily responsible for the emotional symptoms, whilst deficiencies in noradrenaline correlate with the biological symptoms.

Antidepressant drug treatment

Individuals with mild depression are unlikely to benefit from antidepressant medication, whilst those with mild-to-moderate depression they may be more effectively treated by non-drug approaches, such as cognitive-behaviour therapy and exercise. Therapeutic approaches are indicated for moderate to severe major depressive disorder, but still the response to treatment will be greater if combined with the non-drug approaches.

Unipolar depression – drug treatment

The main types of antidepressant drugs used for the management of unipolar depression are discussed in the following sub-sections.

Serotonin and noradrenaline reuptake inhibitors (SNRIs):

The group of medications referred to as serotonin and noradrenaline reuptake inhibitors, such as duloxetine have become the most commonly prescribed antidepressants. Their mode of therapeutic action is similar to TCAs but with a significantly improved side-effect profile.

Side effects with these agents include xerostomia, nausea, sweating, constipation, anorexia, altered sleep patterns (including insomnia and tiredness), and sexual dysfunction.

Selective serotonin reuptake inhibitors (SSRIs):

The SSRIs include drugs such as fluoxetine and citalopram. In general, the SSRIs provide a reasonable balance between effectiveness and side effects.

Side effects associated with SSRI use are nausea, anorexia, insomnia and loss of libido. Unlike TCAs, SSRIs generally do not produce sedation, which renders them less dangerous than TCAs if a patient overdoses. SSRIs are considered to be as effective as TCAs for moderate depression, but probably not as effective for severe depression.

Tricyclic antidepressants (TCAs):

Tricyclic antidepressant drugs, such as amitriptyline and dosulepin, were some of the first effective antidepressant agents, but their use has declined with the advent of newer antidepressant medications with reduced side effect profiles. However, they can be prescribed for managing neuropathic pain (Chapter 6). TCAs inhibit the reuptake of both noradrenaline and serotonin to a similar degree, which is considered to confer their ability to manage both the biological (noradrenaline) and emotional (serotonin) symptoms of depression.

In addition to inhibiting monoamine reuptake, most TCAs block one or more neurotransmitter receptors, including muscarinic acetylcholine receptors, histamine receptors and serotonin receptors. The antagonism of the muscarinic receptors produces the atropine-like side effects, including xerostomia, problems with near-vision, constipation and urinary retention. Another common side effect with TCAs is sedation, caused by antagonism of the histamine H_1 receptor, which can lead to drowsiness.

In contrast to newer antidepressants, TCAs are dangerous in overdose, where they may cause potentially fatal ventricular arrhythmias through elongation of the Q-T interval. However, even clinical doses of TCAs produce a slight increase in the risk of sudden cardiac death.

Noradrenaline reuptake inhibitors (NARIs):

The noradrenaline reuptake inhibitors primarily exert their effect by selectively inhibiting the reuptake of noradrenaline. There is no specific indication regarding the potential interaction with vasoconstrictor-containing local anaesthetics, but it would be appropriate for care to be exercised.

St John's wort (Hypericum):

St John's wort (*Hypericum perforatum*) is a natural medicinal herb remedy, commonly used to manage the symptoms of depression. Importantly, St John's wort has the potential to cause significant drug–drug interactions.

Noradrenaline-serotonin specific antidepressants (NaSSAs):

The noradrenaline-serotonin specific antidepressants, primarily represented by the drug mirtazapine, have become relatively popular. It produces its effect by enhancing noradrenaline and serotonin activity. Mirtazapine also antagonizes the H_1 histamine receptor, which results in a sedative action.

Other agents that exert an antagonist action of presynaptic monoamine receptors include mianserin and trazodone. Xerostomia, headaches and nausea are the more common side effects.

Monoamine oxidase inhibitors (MAOIs):

Monoamine oxidase inhibitors represent one of the first, effective antidepressant medications, but their use has been largely superseded on the grounds of both efficacy and side-effect profile.

The older, non-selective agents can cause significant interactions with foodstuffs, particularly mature cheese, salami and yeast extracts, which contain large amounts of the amino acid, tyramine ('cheese reaction'). However newer, selective agents, such as moclobemide, do not exhibit this effect.

Antidepressant medication effects on oral health and patient care in the clinic:

The most common issue that needs to be managed is xerostomia. While SSRIs have less of an impact on salivary flow than some other antidepressants, some studies indicate that xerostomia is still a potential concern.

Another common issue is postural hypotension. Postural hypotension, will increase the risk of a patient feeling faint when arising from a supine position in the dental chair. These effects will be exacerbated in cases where patients are also being prescribed antihypertensive medications.

For antidepressants that influence serotonin activity, there is a low, but none-the-less important risk of increased bleeding or bruising. Serotonin is an important mediator of normal platelet function and haemostasis, and therapies such as SSRIs and SNRIs may lead to reduced serotonin levels in platelets, and impaired haemostasis. This risk may be increased when non-steroidal anti-inflammatory drugs (NSAIDs) are used concomitantly.

Some antidepressants, particularly TCAs and the NASSA, mirtazapine, can produce sedation due to antagonism of the histamine H_1 receptor. This can lead to drowsiness and difficulties in concentrating. This sedating effect needs to be taken into consideration when using other agents that also exert a centrally mediated depressant effect, such as benzo-diazepines and opioid analgesics.

Due care needs to be exercised when using vasoconstrictor-containing local anaesthetic preparations for patients being prescribed antidepressants, and particularly TCAs. TCAs can potentiate the effects of adrenaline and noradrenaline. The potentiation of adrenaline's effects (~3-fold) is less than for noradrenaline (~8-fold).

While the use of local anaesthetics containing catecholamine vasoconstrictors is not totally contraindicated, due caution needs to be exercised in terms of both the amount of vasoconstrictor administered, and the injection technique.

One of the concerns for patients taking MAOIs is the potential for a hypertensive crisis. However, while they were once considered to be contraindicated, it is now viewed that adrenaline-containing local anaesthetics in dentistry do not pose a significant risk for patients taking MAOIs.

The potential for drug–drug interactions must be taken into consideration with antidepressant medication, particularly with TCAs, MAOIs and St John's wort. For safety reasons, it is essential that St John's wort is discontinued 2 weeks prior to general anaesthesia.

Bipolar disorder – drug treatment

Bipolar disorder is a condition distinct from unipolar depression. The medications prescribed for unipolar depression are not, at least as monotherapies, approved for bipolar disorder. Medical management of bipolar disorder is primarily aimed at stabilizing the condition. Long-term management is more likely to impact upon clinical dental practice.

Drugs used to stabilize bipolar disorder include lithium and some antiepileptic medications. When these agents are used for this condition, they are referred to as mood-stabilizing drugs. In addition, some antipsychotic drugs may also have a role to play in the management of the condition.

Lithium:

The use of lithium is declining, primarily due to its narrow therapeutic window, and toxic effects.

Non-steroidal anti-inflammatory drugs, and the antibiotic, metronidazole, will decrease lithium clearance and increase the risk of lithium toxicity. As such, NSAIDs are best avoided unless essential.

Antiepileptic medications as mood stabilizers:

A number of antiepileptic drugs, including lamotrigine and valproate, are effective in the management of bipolar disorder, and are safer than lithium. They have a slightly higher efficacy in terms of preventing the depressive episodes as compared to the mania.

Side effects are xerostomia, dizziness, headaches, nausea and blurred vision. Patients on chronic medication may have blood dyscrasias, and the potential for bleeding and poor wound healing. For patients on valproate, this may be exacerbated by NSAIDs and aspirin use. Macrolide antibiotics should be avoided for patients on valproate due to their ability to decrease valproate metabolism.

Antipsychotic medications in bipolar disorder:

The antipsychotic medications used to manage bipolar disorder are classified as atypical antipsychotics, and include olanzapine, aripiprazole, risperidone and quetiapine. In general, they are more effective in preventing the manic episodes. These drugs may be given in combination with valproate or lithium in order to provide an effective control over both manic and depressive episodes.

Xersostomia is a side effect of these agents, and they may potentiate the atropine-like effects of other medications. These medications may also enhance the sedative effects of other medications, including the benzodiazepines. In addition, vasoconstrictor-containing local anaesthetics should be used with care due to the potential for increased effects. It is not uncommon for these drugs to cause nervousness, agitation and potentially hostile behaviour.

Table 13.3 lists important points to consider in dental practice with regard to depression.

Anxiety disorders

Anxiety represents another common mood, or affective disorder. Like depression, anxiety represents a normal, emotional response, and care must be taken to distinguish between what represents a natural response, and when it becomes of clinical concern.

The distinction is made when anxiety starts to interfere with a person's normal activities, such as avoiding dental therapy. Anxiety disorders are considered to be very common, and may affect as many as 15% of the population.

There is evidence that severe or long-lasting stress may lead to the changes in the brain associated with anxiety disorders. Anxiety may also be triggered by a significant, traumatic event.

Symptoms include shortness of breath, tachycardia or palpitations, possibly with chest pains, feeling hot or cold, and sweating, feeling dizzy, dry mouth, muscle tension, problems sleeping and gastrointestinal upsets. Anxiety disorders fall into a number of basic categories, discussed in the following sub-sections.

Generalized anxiety disorder

This form of anxiety disorder is characterized by prolonged, excessive worry that cannot be easily controlled by the individual. Generalized anxiety disorder can be effectively treated with benzodiazepines, while other effective medications

---

Table 13.3 Practice points – depression

- The inflammatory basis of depression suggests that poor oral health may be one risk factor for the development of depression.
- Patients with depression may be more prone to poor oral health due to oral health practices, avoidance of routine therapy and poor lifestyle choices.
- Most antidepressant medications cause some degree of xerostomia.
- Care should be exercised in terms of the use of vasoconstrictor-containing local anaesthetics, particularly for patients prescribed TCAs.
- There are a number of potential drug interactions: an increased risk of bleeding with SSRIs and NSAIDs; enhanced sedative effects with TCAs and benzodiazepines; and increased risk of lithium toxicity with NSAIDs.
- Orthostatic hypotension may occur with antidepressant medications.
- Patients with depression may have a reduced pain tolerance.
- Aesthetic dentistry may help patients with depression by enhancing self-esteem, and reducing a sense of ugliness.

may include antidepressants (SSRIs etc) and beta-blockers.

Panic disorder

Panic disorder is a common condition, affecting approximately 2% of the population, at some point in their lives. The physical signs are those associated with sympathetic activity, while the emotional symptoms include a sense of impending doom, fear of death, and a detachment from reality. These attacks commonly last between 15 and 30 minutes. For more than half of sufferers, panic disorder coexists with unipolar depression.

The neurotransmitters serotonin and noradrenaline may play a role in the condition. Another neurotransmitter which has been linked to the disorder is γ-aminobutyric acid (GABA), the main inhibitory neurotransmitter in the brain, Drugs that are able to enhance the effects of GABA, such as the benzodiazepines, are beneficial in managing the problem, although the potential for dependency limits their clinical value.

Therapeutic agents are best combined with cognitive and behavioural therapy. If panic disorder is not appropriately managed, there is the potential for sufferers to develop phobias, particularly agoraphobia.

Phobias

Phobias occur when individuals develop very strong fears of particular situations or objects, such as snakes, spiders, open spaces (agoraphobia), heights, flying and dentists. Commonly, the sufferer will actually be aware that their response is either excessive or irrational, but they are not able to control these emotions.

Obsessive-compulsive disorder

Like panic disorder, obsessive-compulsive disorder is a common condition, affecting around 2% of the population. There appears to be a familial trait. The condition is characterized by obsessions, which are repeated thoughts, and compulsions, which are repeated acts. The aim of the compulsions is to try to reduce the anxiety, which, for the sufferer, is linked to the obsession. One common obsession and compulsion is a fear of infection, combined with excessive, ritualized hand washing. However, dental manifestations are not uncommon, with gingival and dental abrasion associated with excessive oral hygiene practices.

Social anxiety disorder

Social anxiety disorder (SAD) is one of the most common psychological issues, and it frequently begins during the teenage years. The sufferer develops a persistent fear of being scrutinized or judged by others, and they become anxious when they are exposed to their feared social situation.

Treatment of social anxiety disorder is best managed through medical management in combination with behavioural and cognitive therapies.

Post-traumatic stress disorder

While related to anxiety, post-traumatic stress disorder is considered a separate condition. It represents a severe psychiatric disorder that is linked to a traumatic life event. Common symptoms include re-experiencing the event in the form of flashbacks if the sufferer is awake, or nightmares when asleep.

Treatment of PTSD primarily involves psychotherapy, although this may be supplemented by medication.

Anxiety and the dental patient

In general, patients with anxiety disorders may have oral health issues, and concerns about dental visits. Patients with diagnosed anxiety may have xerostomia associated with their anxiolytic medications. In addition, a desire for comfort eating may lead to a diet that is high in cariogenic foods. Oral hygiene practices may be poor even in a person with an obsession for cleanliness.

Dental phobia is one of the most common of all phobias. The problem may be more akin to post-traumatic stress disorder as, unlike many anxiety conditions where the sufferer realizes that their concerns are irrational or excessive, for many individuals with dental phobia there is some ground to their fears.

As many as 75% of the adult population experience some degree of dental fear. However, approximately 5% to 10% of the population are considered to experience dental phobia. These patients are so fearful of receiving dental treatment that they avoid dental care at all costs, often establishing a 'cycle of avoidance'. As such, it is essential that dental fears are managed appropriately in order to prevent this situation from developing.

Anxiolytic medication

An anxiolytic is a drug that is used to treat the symptoms of anxiety. Currently there are a number of different medical approaches that can be used for the management of anxiety.

Antidepressant drugs:

In general, antidepressants are relatively effective agents for the management of most forms of anxiety. The most commonly used agents are the SSRIs and SNRIs, and they allow for the chronic management of the condition.

Benzodiazepines and related sedatives:

Sedatives are drugs that produce sedation. However, in low doses, the same agents are capable of reducing anxiety. Anxiolytics and sedatives are valuable in dental practice, from helping to manage dental anxiety to inducing a state of conscious sedation for dental surgery.

Benzodiazepines are very effective anxiolytic agents, but their potential for tolerance and dependence limits their long-term use for managing anxiety. As such, they are primarily prescribed for the short-term relief of severe and disabling anxiety, as well as being a first choice when short-term CNS sedation is required. The benzodiazepines most commonly used in dentistry are diazepam, temazepam and midazolam.

In general, benzodiazepines basically share the same pharmacological actions, namely that they potentiate the activity of the main inhibitory neurotransmitter in the brain, γ-aminobutyric acid (GABA).

Atypical antipsychotic medications with anxiolytic actions:

Historically, antipsychotic medications, used to manage schizophrenia, have been referred to as 'major tranquilizers', giving some indication of a potential action in anxiety. There is an interest in the use of agents, such as quetiapine and risperidone, as anxiolytics for generalized anxiety disorder, particularly in patients who have not responded to first-line therapies.

Beta-adrenergic receptor antagonists (beta-blockers):

Beta-blockers are drugs that antagonize the actions of adrenaline and noradrenaline on the beta-subtypes of the adrenergic receptors. The physical, or systemic, symptoms of anxiety, such as tachycardia, palpitations, muscle tremors and blushing, occur due to a sympathetic response. Beta-blockers may help to manage these physical signs of anxiety. Beta-blockers are primarily used to help manage social anxiety and performance anxiety, such as public speaking. They are contraindicated in patents with obstructive respiratory conditions, such as asthma. In the dental clinic, orthostatic hypotension may occur and patients should be seated after lying supine.

CHAPTER 14

Central nervous system 2 – neurodegenerative and acquired disorders

Alan Nimmo

Key Topics

- Introduction to neurodegenerative and acquired brain disorders
- Strokes, and their impact on oral hygiene and oral health
- Neurodegenerative disorders and their impact on oral health
- Multiple sclerosis

Learning Objectives

- Be aware of the impacts that acquired and neurodegenerative brain disorders may have upon oral hygiene and oral health
- Be aware of the importance of good preventive care for patients with acquired and neurodegenerative brain disorders
- Be aware of the importance in involving caregivers in order to improve patients' oral hygiene and oral health
- Be aware of the care that needs to be exercised in terms of managing these patients in the dental clinic

Essential Dental Therapeutics, First Edition. Edited by David Wray.
© 2018 John Wiley & Sons Ltd. Published 2018 by John Wiley & Sons Ltd.
Companion Website: www.wiley.com/go/wray/dental-therapeutics

Introduction

Given optimal conditions, the human brain can function very effectively for over 100 years. However, in order to achieve this, the delicate neurons need to be physically and functionally protected. Physical protection of the brain is provided by the bony cranium, the meningeal membranes, as well as the buoyancy afforded by the cerebrospinal fluid. In addition, the cerebrospinal fluid, together with the blood-brain barrier, provides a very protected, stable environment for neuronal function. The brain also receives approximately 20% of cardiac output, ensuring a constant supply of blood glucose and oxygen to meet its high metabolic demands. Finally, the central nervous system has its own, dedicated immune protection, provided by microglia, to deal with injury and infection. Failure of any of these protective mechanisms can lead to permanent brain damage and associated functional deficits. Acquired brain damage as a result of a stroke is unfortunately a common issue. Strokes represent the third-leading cause of death, but equally significant is the fact that they are the leading cause of adult disability. Deficits that impact on motor function can have direct effects on the ability of sufferers to perform basic oral hygiene practices.

Neurodegenerative disorders, such as Alzheimer's disease and Parkinson's disease, also represent a growing concern, particularly with our aging populations. While, as with cancer, increasing age is a risk factor for their development, it is not, in itself, a cause. Although there is still much to learn about the pathological mechanisms underlying neurodegenerative disorders, the mis-folding of proteins during their synthesis, and the subsequent aggregation of insoluble proteins, does appear to be an important, common mechanism. However, there is also evidence that inflammation, and particularly chronic neuroinflammation, also plays a role in neurodegenerative processes.

The disorders, Huntingdon's disease, motor neurone disease and multiple sclerosis will also be considered in turn.

In relation to oral health, much of the impact of these disorders is due to their effect on oral hygiene practices, although there may also be issues around medication, and patient management in the dental clinic. Dental professionals may also need to work collaboratively with these patients' carers in order to achieve the best oral-health outcomes.

Stroke

A stroke, or cerebrovascular accident, is associated with an interruption of the blood supply to a region of the brain that results in an infarction, or neuronal death, in the affected area. Normal cerebral perfusion can be interrupted in a number of different ways. The most common mechanism is a thrombotic event within a cerebral artery. Thrombotic strokes are frequently associated with the development of an atherosclerotic plaque in a cerebral artery. The plaque causes narrowing, and eventual occlusion of a vessel due to thrombus formation, particularly if the plaque ruptures. Strokes may also occur as a result of an embolism. Embolic strokes commonly involve blood clot, or thrombus, fragments that have formed outside of the brain, and travel to the brain through the circulation. Once in the cerebral circulation, they may occlude a cerebral vessel, commonly at a site of vessel bifurcation or narrowing. By their nature, the onset of embolic strokes is always very sudden and can involve very large regions of brain. Predisposing factors for embolic strokes include atrial fibrillation, bacterial endocarditis, and heart valve disease. Together, thrombotic and embolic strokes are referred to as ischaemic strokes, and account for more than 80% of all cerebrovascular accidents.

Other cerebrovascular accidents are associated with haemorrhage. Haemorrhagic strokes, also known as intracerebral haemorrhages, are most commonly caused by uncontrolled hypertension leading to weakening, and subsequent rupture of a blood vessel. Haemorrhagic strokes most commonly occur in deeper brain structures, particularly in the region of the basal ganglia.

A very severe headache is a consistent finding, while other symptoms depend upon the region affected. The release of blood from the ruptured vessel can cause further ischaemia in the brain, as a result of cerebral vasospasm.

A subarachnoid haemorrhage, where there is bleeding in the subarachnoid space of the meningeal membranes, can also cause a stroke. The rupture of a vessel is most commonly associated with the presence of an aneurysm, which weakens the vessel wall, although subarachnoid haemorrhages may also occur with head injuries. The risk of an aneurysm rupturing is exacerbated by uncontrolled hypertension.

The mechanisms associated with ischaemic strokes can also give rise to transient ischaemic attacks (TIAs). In some cases, the obstructing clot can be efficiently removed by the body's fibrinolytic system before any permanent tissue damage occurs. As a result, the early symptoms of the 'stroke' can resolve without evidence of neurologic dysfunction. However, these signs should not be ignored, since TIAs are an important warning sign of cerebrovascular disease, and sufferers carry a high risk of a subsequent stroke.

The signs and symptoms of a stroke will vary depending upon the vessel, and with that, the area of the brain affected. The initial signs of a stroke normally comprise a mixture of motor and sensory impairment. Motor impairment may result in weakness or clumsiness on one side of the body, along with difficulties in swallowing, slurred speech, and double vision. There may also be problems with language comprehension, balance and vision, as well as somatosensory loss.

It is important to be aware of the signs of a stroke, since early clinical intervention is critical. The acronym FAST (**F**acial weakness; **A**rm weakness; **S**peech problems; **T**ime to call) has been proposed as an easy mechanism for assessment. Early detection and intervention with a stroke is critical, although therapeutic management is limited. Early identification of an ischaemic stroke can allow for the administration of the tissue plasminogen activator (tPA), alteplase, to remove the clot. However, most therapeutic intervention for stroke is aimed at prevention.

Since the majority of strokes are triggered by either a blood clot, or clot fragment, prevention of thrombus formation is a cornerstone of prevention. Depending on stroke risk, patients may either be prescribed antiplatelet (e.g. aspirin, clopidogrel) or anticoagulant (e.g. warfarin, dabigatrin) medication. Obviously, the potential for excessive bleeding needs to be managed within the dental clinic. However, this must be achieved by the use of local

measures rather than the cessation of anticoagulant or antiplatelet therapy.

As mentioned, hypertension is an important risk factor for both ischaemic and haemorrhagic strokes. As such, good control of blood pressure reduces the incidence of strokes. A variety of antihypertensive agents may be used, including diuretics, ACE inhibitors, calcium channel blockers and beta-blockers. In terms of oral health, the main issue is the potential for xerostomia with these agents. Unlike with cardiovascular disease, the link between cholesterol and stroke is not as clear cut, but large clinical trials have shown that statin therapy may reduce the incidence of strokes in high-risk patients. Whilst statins provide some benefit in high-risk patients, both antiplatelet and antihypertensive drugs are about twice as effective for stroke prevention.

Recovery from a stroke depends upon the size and location of infarct. Rehabilitation is a critical element of the recovery process, and should begin as early as possible. However, even with rehabilitation, many patients will have residual deficits.

Impact on oral hygiene and oral health

The dental profession has an active role to play in the management of stroke sufferers from the rehabilitation phase onwards. It is quite common for a stroke to have a direct impact on the oral cavity. For some, basic functions such as eating, drinking, swallowing and speech, may be impaired. Facial palsy is also a common issue.

Effective communication with stroke victims is a key part of care provision. A significant number of sufferers will have deficits that impact on speech and communication (aphasia and dysarthria). These problems are not reflective of a loss of intelligence, but rather an impaired capacity to articulate their thoughts and feelings. The impairment may be linked to a reduced ability to process language, or simply reduced control over the muscles involved in speech production. As such, good communication skills on the part of the care provider are essential.

There are a number of issues that can impact upon oral health in stroke victims. To begin with, many of the risk factors for strokes, such as smoking and poor diet, are common contributors to poor oral health. Following a stroke, the motor and sensory impairment can cause food debris to accumulate, particularly on the affected side. Dietary adjustments following a stroke may also pose an increased risk for caries.

Maintenance of oral and denture hygiene is an important aspect of stroke management, and the basic principles are the same as for all members of society. However, stroke sufferers may have muscle weakness, loss of dexterity, and loss of sensation, all of which impact on the ability to undertake self-care, particularly if the stroke affects their dominant hand. Good oral hygiene is also particularly important for patients with dysphagia. In many cases, good oral hygiene may be dependent upon the support of a carer, either personal or professional. Strokes may also impact upon the ability of a patient to cope with treatment in the dental clinic, and care should be taken to make the patient comfortable.

Neurodegenerative disorders

As mentioned previously, neurodegenerative disorders are of growing concern, particularly with our aging populations. There are a number of different neurodegenerative disorders, such as Alzheimer's and Parkinson's disease. As the name suggests, a common element of these conditions is the neuronal loss, and associated dysfunction. The mis-folding and accumulation of abnormal proteins is also a common feature associated with these conditions. However, different neurodegenerative disorders can affect different areas and pathways of the brain, so there must also be different disease mechanisms. In some conditions the neurodegeneration primarily affects cognitive and memory function, leading to the dementia associated with conditions such as Alzheimer's disease. In others, there may be more impact on motor function, as seen with Parkinson's disease and Huntington's chorea. However, both forms of neurodegeneration may adversely impact upon oral health, and also pose special issues in terms of providing care within the clinic.

Alzheimer's disease

Alzheimer's disease represents the most common form of both neurodegeneration and dementia.

While age is not a cause, there is a strong correlation between increased age and increased incidence of the condition. As such, dentists are likely to have an increased proportion of patients who suffer from dementia, and therefore an understanding of the issues posed can help improve the quality of life of the sufferers. While the cause of Alzheimer's is unknown, there is increasing evidence for an underlying inflammatory component, and this may lead to a relationship with periodontal disease.

There are certain characteristic changes associated with Alzheimer's disease, although these do not fully explain the development of the condition. In terms of histopathology, two characteristics are the presence of deposits of β-amyloid proteins (amyloid plaques) and neurofibrillary tangles, associated with over-phosphorylation of a neuronal protein, tau. At the gross level, there is atrophy of the cerebral cortex. However, there is some specificity to the neurodegenerative changes. Acetylcholine-containing nerves, particularly those associated with the hippocampus and frontal cortex, appear to be most affected. These changes may underlie the impact of Alzheimer's on both short-term memory and cognitive function. The specific impact on cholinergic transmission also provides a target for therapeutic management.

Currently, the therapeutic management of Alzheimer's disease is aimed at slowing the progression of the condition, primarily through increasing acetylcholine levels in the brain. These treatments may be beneficial in the early and moderate stages of the disease, but their beneficial effects are limited. The main agents used in Alzheimer's are acetylcholinesterase inhibitors (e.g. donepezil (Aricept), galantamine (Razadyne) and rivastigmine (Exelon)) which reduce the breakdown of acetylcholine, thereby increasing its activity. The main side effects of these agents reflect the increased levels of acetylcholine in the body, and may include nausea, vomiting and diarrhoea.

Oral health care:

Individuals with Alzheimer's disease are at risk of poor, and rapidly declining oral health. Much of this is directly related to the condition. Dental or denture hygiene practices are omitted, as patients first start to forget to carry these out, and eventually forget how to perform oral hygiene. Patients may also loose manual dexterity. These problems may be compounded by the side effects of the patient's medication, particularly if they cause xerostromia.

The management of patients with Alzheimer's requires a high level of communication skills, allied to careful clinical management. That clinical management will be easiest in the early stages of the condition, and therefore one should aim at performing any major treatment during this stage. As for all patients, good preventive care is essential, including managing problems such as xerostomia. In terms of oral hygiene, it is good to encourage patients to be independent, but it is also beneficial to educate the carers in supervising and assisting with these practices. As their condition progresses, patients will have more of a problem comprehending what is happening to them, increasing the feelings of agitation and anxiety in the clinic, and therefore appointments should be kept as short, and as stress-free as possible.

As indicated, currently the main therapeutic approach to the management of Alzheimer's is increasing acetylcholine activity through the use of cholinesterase inhibitors. Since acetylcholine is the main neurotransmitter associated with salivary gland function, there is a tendency to hypersalivation (sialorrhoea), which may pose challenges for dental treatment. Unfortunately, as far as dental health is concerned, the tendency for these drugs to also cause nausea and vomiting can still predispose sufferers to acid erosion. As is more common with medications, the adjunctive therapies, such as anti-depressant medication, is more likely to cause xerostomia.

Within the clinic, anxiolytics and sedatives, such as benzodiazepines, may be used to reduce patient agitation and improve cooperation. However, care must be exercised to avoid over sedation if the patient is taking other medications that have a CNS-depressant effect, such as the antipsychotic, haloperidol, or tricyclic antidepressants. Alzheimer's patients are unlikely to be candidates for inhaled sedation, as they are unlikely to tolerate the nasal hood. In terms of analgesia, patients prescribed cholinesterase inhibitors have a greater risk of gastric irritation and ulceration with NSAIDs, since

cholinesterase inhibitors increase gastric acid secretion. There are other potential drug–drug interactions to be aware of with cholinesterase inhibitors. Some antimicrobial agents, including erythromycin and ketoconazole, can decrease the metabolism of cholinesterase inhibitors, leading to excessive acetylcholine activity.

Parkinson's disease

Parkinson's disease is a progressive neurodegenerative disorder that primarily impacts upon the central control of movement. In this condition the neuronal loss is primarily associated with the dopamine-containing nerves of the substantia nigra that form a pathway from the midbrain to the corpus striatum of the basal ganglia. This pathway is critical in terms of producing smooth, coordinated voluntary movement, and loss of function leads to impaired motor function. However, neuronal loss is not just confined to this pathway, but may have wider impacts in the brain, resulting in depression, dementia and autonomic dysfunction.

The primary signs of Parkinson's disease relate to the loss of normal, voluntary motor control. Muscle tremors normally begin to appear in the hand, with an involuntary 'pill rolling' movement, but then may spread to the legs, face, tongue and jaw. There may be difficulty in initiating voluntary movements, a problem referred to as bradykinesia. This is partly due to muscle rigidity, but is also related to inertia within the central motor control pathways. The other side of this coin is, that once movement has started, it is also harder to stop. There is a general increase in muscle tension, and this rigidity results in an increased resistance to passive movement. The loss of motor control impacts on posture and gait. Sufferers tend to walk with a rather stooped posture, and take short shuffling steps. There is also a reduction in facial expressions, potentially resulting in a 'mask-like' appearance. Autonomic dysfunction is also common, with perhaps the most significant issue for the dental clinic being postural hypotension. Other problems may include depression, and less commonly, the development of dementia.

Since Parkinson's disease is primarily associated with a loss of dopaminergic neurotransmission, the primary approach to treatment is to increase dopamine activity in the brain. The first line of treatment is levodopa, which is a precursor for dopamine synthesis

Oral impacts of Parkinson's disease:

There are a number of aspects associated with Parkinson's disease that impact upon oral health and oral care. The problem of dysphagia, together with dietary adjustments to manage it, such as high levels of refined carbohydrates, significantly impacts upon oral health. As a dental practitioner it is important not to give conflicting and confusing advice, but instead work with the medical team to improve oral health.

Naturally, the poor motor control impacts upon oral hygiene practices. It is important to support independent care as much as possible, for example through the use of electric toothbrushes, but the support of a carer may be required to help with oral hygiene. Oral hygiene may be supplemented by fluoride and chlorhexidine-containing preparations, but agents that could be aspirated, due to their dysphagia, such as mouthwash, should be avoided. The patient's reduced motor control may also impact upon their ability to wear dentures.

In the dental clinic, appointments should be as short and stress-free as possible in order to not exacerbate their problems. The patient may require physical assistance to get in and out of the dental chair. Effective suction is also important during procedures in order to prevent aspiration.

Huntington's disease

Huntington's disease is an inherited condition that results in progressive, rapid neuronal degeneration. It is associated with severe jerky, involuntary motor movements, particularly affecting the fingers, face and tongue, along with progressive dementia. It appears to be associated with loss of γ-aminobutyric acid (GABA) inhibitory activity. Approaches to controlling the symptoms include drugs that decrease dopamine activity (e.g. tetrabenazine, chlorpromazine) or increase GABA activity (benzodiazepines, baclofen).

The principles of preventive oral care, such as fluoride treatment, and oral hygiene are the same as for all patients. Good preventive care is the cornerstone of managing oral health in Huntington's disease. Given the inherited nature of the condition, good oral care should be provided before the onset of the symptoms to provide the best outcomes. Once symptoms begin, the ability to perform oral hygiene is affected, but may be aided by an electric toothbrush. As with Parkinson's, dysphagia is a problem, and sufferers may also have difficulty wearing dentures. If there is recurrent lip trauma caused by movements, a mouthguard may have a protective effect. Involuntary movements are also an issue in the dental clinic, but treatment may be assisted by conscious sedation, particularly given the fact that drugs which increase GABA activity, such as benzodiazepines, help to control the symptoms of Huntington's.

Motor neuron disease

Motor neuron disease (MND) is a term that covers a group of neurodegenerative conditions that affect the upper motor neurons of the cerebral cortex, and the lower motor neurons of the brain stem and spinal cord. MND normally has a rapid progression (median life expectancy following diagnosis is 3 years), and is universally fatal due to the loss of respiratory muscle function and associated respiratory failure. It most commonly begins by affecting the limbs, although the muscles of the mouth and throat may also be involved early in the disease, leading to dysphagia and drooling, along with the risk of aspiration. Currently medical management is primarily symptomatic, although riluzole, an inhibitor of glutamate release, may be used to reduce the toxic effects of the neurotransmitter glutamate, and slow neurodegeneration. From an oral perspective, the main side effects of riluzole are a risk of nausea and vomiting.

Given the nature of the disease, it may be expected to impact upon oral health due to dysphagia, a reduced capacity for independent oral hygiene practices, nutritional adaptations, and problems in terms of physical access to dental care facilities.

Multiple sclerosis

Multiple sclerosis (MS) is a chronic inflammatory condition that leads to the demyelination of neurons in the brain and spinal cord. This results in both motor and sensory disturbances, and may manifest symptoms of orofacial pain. The precise cause of the condition is unknown, but there is a complex interaction between genetic factors, environmental factors, and potentially infective agents, such as the Epstein-Barr virus. The condition combines both inflammatory and neurodegenerative components.

In terms of treatment, a combination of disease-modifying therapies and symptomatic therapy may be used. Disease-modifying therapies include agents such as interferon-β, which have an immunomodulatory action, and down-regulate the inflammatory response. Symptomatic relief may be obtained by drugs that mimic (e.g. baclofen) or enhance GABA activity (e.g. benzodiazepines). These agents, along with anticonvulsants (e.g. carbamazepine or gabapentin) and tricyclic antidepressants can help manage muscle spasms and associated pain. Analgesia may also be required for additional pain relief.

In terms of dental care, it is important to be aware that common symptoms include orofacial pain, numbness and muscle spasms. The pain is primarily neuropathic in origin, and trigeminal neuralgia occurs in up to 5% of MS patients and may be the presenting symptom. Patients presenting with trigeminal neuralgia should have MS excluded as a cause, especially in younger patients. Oral health may be affected by reduced motor skills impacting on oral hygiene, as well as difficulties in attending dental clinics as the disease progresses. Dentists also need to be aware of the potential issues with the medications used in the management of MS, including xerostomia, sedation, gingival hyperplasia, and orthostatic hypotension.

CHAPTER 15

Central nervous system 3 – genetic and developmental disorders

Alan Nimmo

Key Topics

- Introduction to psychiatric and neurological disorders
- Seizures and epilepsy
- Schizophrenia
- Cerebral Palsy
- Down syndrome

Learning Objectives

- Be aware of the distinction between seizures and epilepsy
- Be aware of the impact epilepsy, and its management, may have upon oral health and, should the need arise, how to manage seizures in the dental clinic
- Be aware of the impact that conditions such as schizophrenia may have upon oral health, and the importance of good preventive care
- Be aware of the impact of cerebral palsy upon oral health, the importance of preventive care, and the careful management of patients in the dental clinic

Essential Dental Therapeutics, First Edition. Edited by David Wray.
© 2018 John Wiley & Sons Ltd. Published 2018 by John Wiley & Sons Ltd.
Companion Website: www.wiley.com/go/wray/dental-therapeutics

Introduction

Psychiatric and neurological disorders are very common in society, but they are often poorly understood. Unfortunately, individuals with these conditions are more susceptible to systemic disease, and are likely to have poorer oral health than other members of the general population. Individuals with severe mental illness are more likely to have decayed, missing or filled teeth. These individuals should have the same level of access to quality healthcare as all members of society. In order to help bridge this gap, it is important to have an understanding of the common neurological conditions, and the approaches that are taken to help manage these conditions. In this way, we can try to prevent these conditions from becoming a barrier to good general and oral healthcare, and develop strategies for improving oral health.

The central nervous system is the most complex organ system within the human body, and we are only beginning to understand its function, and the conditions that affect it. There are some CNS disorders, such as Huntington's disease (Chapter 12), that are linked to a single gene. Other CNS disorders may have a genetic component that serves as a predisposition to developing a particular condition. Whether one does or not, may depend upon other influences, such as environmental factors. For example, with epilepsy, we all have a certain seizure threshold in our brain (i.e. a tendency to develop seizure activity). Individuals with a low seizure threshold, which appears to have a genetic component, are more predisposed to developing epilepsy than others. However, even identical, or monozygotic, twins, who share identical genetic material, will not necessarily both develop epilepsy. Environmental factors, such as injury or inflammation, may serve as the actual trigger for the development of epilepsy. Other conditions, such as cerebral palsy, may be acquired during brain development. Injury to the brain may occur as the result of insults like infection or hypoxia that occur anytime from *in utero* development through to the early childhood years.

There may be a number of factors that can impact upon oral health. Patients may have poor oral hygiene as a result of neglect, lack of motivation, or reduced physical ability to perform good oral care. A patient's medication may also impact upon their oral health, with xerostomia being a common issue. Patients may have problems accessing health-care facilities, and may require additional support and understanding within the dental clinic. Where appropriate, dental professionals may also need to work collaboratively with a patient's carers in order to achieve the best oral-health outcomes.

Seizures and epilepsy

The term seizure applies to the situation where there is an episode of abnormal electrical activity within the brain, which will disrupt normal neuronal activity, and as such, normal brain function. The precise impact of a seizure will depend upon where the abnormal activity occurs, and how widespread the disruption is. The site at which the abnormal activity begins is regularly referred to as the focus, but it may subsequently spread to other areas of the brain. While seizures are commonly thought to involve physical convulsions of the sufferer, that is not always the case. Certainly, if the motor cortex is involved, then convulsions will be observed. However, as with strokes, the precise signs and symptoms depend upon the specific area that is affected. For example, if the seizure involves the brain stem, and in particular the reticular formation, then a loss of consciousness may be observed.

Seizures themselves represent a symptom of some underlying neurological disorder. They are thought to occur as a result of altered neuronal excitability, which may occur through changes at the level of the neuronal cell membrane, or an imbalance between normal excitatory (e.g. glutamate) and inhibitory (e.g. γ-aminobutyric acid (GABA)) transmission in the brain. Seizures may be classified as either being provoked or unprovoked. With provoked seizures, the abnormal activity can be clearly linked to some direct underlying cause. For example, seizures may be triggered by a high fever, particularly in children (febrile seizures), or due to hypoxia or hypoglycaemia. These provoked seizures are best dealt with by treating the underlying cause, for example the use of anti-pyretic medication for febrile seizures. With unprovoked seizures, no obvious underlying cause is observed. This type of seizure is primarily associated with the condition of epilepsy.

Epilepsy is the term used to describe conditions where there is an associated risk of repeated episodes of seizure activity. It is a relatively common disorder, affecting between 0.5% and 1% of the population. There is strong evidence for a genetic component to the condition, and a number of genes, particularly ones encoding for neuronal ion channels and neurotransmitter receptors, have been implicated in the development of the condition. However, while heritability is high, environmental factors also have an influence, since just over half of identical twins will both develop the condition.

Both seizures and epileptic seizures are classified according to the location, nature and impact of the seizure activity. The first distinction is to categorize a seizure as being focal or generalized. Focal seizures describe the situation where the abnormal activity, at least to begin with, is relatively localized. Previously, these were more commonly referred to as partial seizures. In some cases a specific brain lesion may be identified as being responsible for the epileptic focus. The precise impact of that seizure will depend upon the region of the brain that is affected. For example if the motor cortex is involved convulsions will be observed.

A generalized seizure refers to the situation where the seizure activity spreads rapidly to involve multiple areas of the brain, including cortical and subcortical structures. Generalized seizures are grouped into a number of classes, with two important groups being tonic-clonic seizures and absence seizures. From a clinical perspective, a tonic-clonic seizure can represent a confronting situation for the clinician. The seizure begins with whole-body muscle spasms that last about a minute, and cause breathing to stop. The patient's face will become blue, unlike a fainting episode, where it normally becomes pale. This is followed by a few minutes of jerking contractions, which gradually phase out. The patient is likely to remain unconscious for a few more minutes, before slowly recovering. When the patient comes round, they are likely to be confused, feel unwell, and require reassurance. Occasionally a patient may experience a series of unremitting seizures, and this situation, referred to as status epilepticus, constitutes a medical emergency (see Chapter 10). Absence seizures, most commonly observed in children, are less dramatic, but may occur more frequently. They are characterized by the sufferer suddenly ceasing what they are doing, for example, stopping speaking mid-sentence, and appearing to be oblivious to their surroundings.

Management of epilepsy

Epilepsy is managed through the use of antiepileptic medications. Antiepileptic medications are primarily symptomatic in their action, helping to reduce the risk of a seizure rather than treating the underlying cause. With careful therapeutic control, the seizure activity can be well managed in approximately 75% of patients. However, some patients will continue to experience regular seizures despite the best therapeutic attempts. Antiepileptic medication primarily reduces excitatory activity through either reducing sodium ion channel activity, reducing calcium ion channel activity, or enhancing the activity of GABA. A number of antiepileptic medications target neuronal action potential generation (e.g. carbamazepine, phenytoin, lamotrigine). There are also a number of effective agents that produce their effects primarily through calcium ion channel activity. These agents include valproate and ethosuxamide, which are primarily used to manage absence seizures, along with gabapentin and pregabalin, which are primarily used for focal seizures. There are number of different ways in which GABA activity can be enhanced. Benzodiazepines and phenobarbital will facilitate the activation of $GABA_A$ receptors. Once seizure control has been achieved, it is important the therapies are carefully maintained in order to prevent break-through seizure activity.

Epilepsy and the dental patient

Although not widely studied, the general consensus is that patients with epilepsy are more likely to have poorer oral health when compared to their non-epileptic counterparts. One reason for this may be a lack of access to quality dental care. The impact on oral health also appears to be related to how well an individual's epilepsy is managed by their medication. If a patient's epilepsy is well controlled, they are likely to display better oral health than those individuals with poor seizure control.

In terms of oral health, all aspects appear to be potentially affected in epilepsy, with increased levels of decayed and missing teeth, and poorer periodontal health. Oral trauma, affecting both soft tissues and the dentition, is also common, particularly in patients who experience tonic-clonic seizures

In general, antiepileptic medications do not have a significant impact on oral health. Perhaps the best-documented effect is the potential for phenytoin to cause gingival hyperplasia. Xerostomia and gingival bleeding have been reported for carbamazepine and valproate, but the newer medications appear to have little in the way of oral side effects.

It is important to be aware that some dentistry-prescribed medications can interact with antiepileptic drugs. Again, problems are more commonly observed with the 'older' antiepileptic agents, phenytoin, carbamazepine and valproate. Some antibacterial and antifungal agents (e.g. metronidazole, erythromycin, and particularly fluconazole) can reduce the metabolism of phenytoin and increase its activity. Clarithromycin has a similar effect on carbamazepine, while aspirin can potentiate the effects of valproate.

While seizures are rare in the dental clinic, it is essential that the dental staff are prepared to provide emergency care if required. If a patient starts to have a seizure, they must be protected from physical injury by quickly clearing all surgical instruments and equipment from the vicinity, and placing the chair in a low, supine position. The patient should be placed on their side to prevent aspiration, but they should not be restrained. The patient should be administered oxygen until they recover. If the patient has repeated fits, or if the fit lasts longer than 5 minutes, then the benzodiazepine, midazolam should be administered into the buccal cavity (10 mg for an adult patient). If a patient has had prolonged or repeated seizures, or this was their first, or an atypical seizure, then an ambulance should be called. For other patients, they should not be allowed to leave the clinic until they are fully recovered. No more dental work should be undertaken on the day, but an oral examination may be performed to check for any injuries. (see also Chapter 10).

Schizophrenia

In Chapter 13, we introduced psychological disorders that impact on the mood of a patient, but do not alter thought processing. In contrast, psychotic disorders, such as schizophrenia, are associated with altered thought processing, or cognition, often in combination with mood swings. Schizophrenia is a common problem, affecting around 1% of the population, with the symptoms normally first appearing around the late teens or early twenties. The terms schizophrenia literally means 'splitting of the mind' which is often 'misinterpreted' as suggesting that the sufferer has a split personality, which is not the case. Instead, the term indicates that the individual may have a problem focussing on the reality of situations. Naturally, one key function of our brain is the ability to 'filter out' insignificant sensory information. This function appears to be impaired in schizophrenia, causing the brain to be 'bombarded' by sensory input, making it difficult for the sufferer to focus on what is important or relevant. As a result, this can cause a detachment from reality.

A wide range of symptoms may be associated with schizophrenia, and these can vary between individuals. Some of the more common indications, referred to as positive symptoms, include delusions and hallucinations, along with disorganized behaviour, thought patterns and motor activity. Delusions refer to the impression that one's actions are controlled by some greater power, while the hallucinations are mainly auditory in nature, with the sufferer 'hearing voices'. The condition leads to a number of negative signs, which include social withdrawal, flattened emotional responses, an inability to experience pleasure, together with feelings of anxiety, guilt and depression. The positive symptoms may be intermittent in nature, but the negative ones are more chronic. As a result, schizophrenia is a very debilitating condition, with high rates of unemployment, homelessness, poor general health and a high risk of attempted suicide.

It is recognized that there may be a strong genetic predisposition to schizophrenia. It is highly polygenic in nature, with more than one hundred putative genes being identified. Environmental factors also play a significant role in the development of the condition, particularly factors that may impact upon brain development. It terms of the functional changes seen in schizophrenia, these are thought to be associated with two main neuronal pathways, the mesolimbic pathway and the mesocortical pathway. Both of these pathways use dopamine as their main neurotransmitter. Much of our understanding, and treatment of schizophrenia is based around dopamine. At the simplest level, drugs that increase dopamine activity can induce schizophrenic-like behaviour. Indeed, one of the side effects levodopa treatment in Parkinson's is hallucinations. In contrast, dopamine antagonists can help control the symptoms of schizophrenia.

There are currently over 40 antipsychotic agents in clinical use, and they can help many sufferers lead more normal lives. These drugs are broadly divided into two groups, first-generation, or typical antipsychotics, and second-generation, or atypical, antipsychotics. The typical antipsychotics include drugs like chlorpromazine and haloperidol. The newer, second-generation antipsychotics, drugs like clozapine, resperidone and quetiapine, have improved efficacy and reduced side effects. Both typical and atypical agents are relatively effective in managing the positive symptoms, while the atypical agents may also help to manage the negative symptoms.

Considerations within the dental clinic

As mentioned earlier, individuals with schizophrenia, as well as other severe mental illnesses, have a tendency to poor overall health, having an increased risk of conditions like type 2 diabetes and cardiovascular disease. In terms of oral health, sufferers are up to three times more likely to be edentulous. The incidence of carious lesions and dental restorations is also significantly increased. There are a number of factors that may be contributing to these issues. The levels of cigarette smoking and substance abuse may be a problem, as is poor dietary choices. Sufferers may have a low motivation to perform oral hygiene practices, and may not be encouraged to do so by their care providers. Access to healthcare facilities may also be an issue. All these issues may be compounded by medication-induced xerostomia, and the other oral side effects associated with antipsychotics.

Effective preventive care, incorporating good oral hygiene practices and prophylactic agents (e.g. artificial saliva, fluoride treatment) is the cornerstone of effective treatment. One of the barriers to preventive care may be the lack of appropriate motivation on the part of the individual. As such, trying to involve a family member or professional care-giver in encouraging oral hygiene may be of significant benefit.

As with all patients, an accurate medical history is vital. If the patient consents, it may also be valuable to consult with their physician in terms of developing their treatment plan. Care must be exercised to prevent the risk of drug interactions with dental medications, particularly for patients prescribed typical antipsychotic agents. One concern is the risk of CNS depression if agents, such as opioid analgesics or benzodiazepines, are used in combination with antipsychotic drugs. Orthostatic hypotension is also a potential concern, so patients should be allowed to rise slowly from the dental chair. Bone marrow suppression, and low leukocyte counts may be an issue, particularly for patients on clozapine, and this must be taken into account when planning dental treatment. The effects of antipsychotic medication on motor control (extrapyramidal symptoms), and the production of Parkinson's-like symptoms, can also impact upon dental treatment, as well as cause an impaired gag reflex.

Attention deficit/hyperactivity disorder

Another condition that appears to be associated with altered dopamine activity in the brain is Attention deficit/hyperactivity disorder (ADHD). As the name suggests this is a condition associated with a pattern of over-activity combined with a limited attention span. These characteristics may have a disruptive effect on both the educational and social development of the children. There has been some controversy over the extent of drug treatment for ADHD, although treatment efficacy has been demonstrated in clinical trials. It is recognized that drug treatment should only be one aspect of patient management following a careful diagnosis.

The drugs prescribed for ADHD are CNS stimulants, and include atomoxetine, a noradrenaline re-uptake inhibitor, and methylphenidate (Ritalin), a noradrenaline and dopamine re-uptake inhibitor. In terms of oral health, the most prominent issue is xerostomia. As a result, good oral hygiene, stimulating saliva production, and the use of saliva substitutes should be encouraged. The cardiovascular effects of these medications are an issue, and therefore due care must be exercised in terms of adrenaline-containing local anaesthetics.

Cerebral palsy

Cerebral palsy occurs as a result of injury to the developing brain, either during foetal development, at birth, or within the first few years of life. Most of these insults (~80%) occur during foetal development, with common causes being maternal infection, hypoxia or hypotension. The effect of the insults is a permanent, but not progressive brain injury. The prevalence of cerebral palsy is around 0.3% of live births. With the heterogeneous nature of the insults and their timings, the term cerebral palsy covers a broad group of conditions. These are primarily associated with movement disorders, but may also be accompanied by altered sensory and cognitive function as well. Epilepsy is also more common in individuals with cerebral palsy.

The impact of cerebral palsy on limb movement is classified as being unilateral or bilateral. The most common form of the condition is referred to as spastic cerebral palsy, where increased muscle tone (hypertonia) results in stiff, jerky movements. Less common are the dyskinetic and ataxic forms of the condition. The motor disturbances with dyskinesia include repetitive twisting movements (dystonia) and unpredictable irregular movements (chorea). Least common is the ataxic form, which is associated with clumsy, uncoordinated movements. There is also a significant variation in the severity or degree of motor impairment, ranging from being able to walk and run, but with some reduction in balance and coordination, through to no capacity for independent mobility.

The management of cerebral palsy will normally involve a range of healthcare professionals, including physiotherapists and occupational therapsts, as well as physicians. Medical treatment is primarily

symptomatic, and is aimed at reducing muscle tone. Muscle tone may be reduced by enhancing GABA activity, for example through the use of benzodiazepines (e.g. diazepam), baclofen (intrathecal) and gabapentin. Botulinum toxin A injections may also be used to give localized relief from muscle spasm.

Considerations within the dental clinic

Cerebral palsy is associated with a broad range of oral and dental issues. Common issues include malocclusion, bruxism and temporomandibular joint disorders. The incidence of traumatic dental injury may also be higher in this population. The incidence of caries is high in individuals with cerebral palsy, and this may be due to a combination of poor oral hygiene practices associated with impaired motor control, diet, and the impact of dysphagia. Dysphagia is more commonly an issue in children with moderate to severe cerebral palsy. Drooling is also a problem, and is primarily due to poor swallowing associated with oral-motor dysfunction.

As for all patients, good preventive care is paramount. For cerebral palsy this may require a caregiver taking an active role in helping to maintain good oral hygiene, and this may be supplemented by dietary improvement. Within the clinic, uncontrolled muscle activity is the primary concern, both for the patient and the clinician's well being. Care must be taken to position and support the patient carefully, and mouth props may be required. Conscious sedation may aid clinical work, although not all patients will tolerate the nasal hood for inhaled sedation. If used, care must be taken with sedation, since most of the agents used for managing cerebral palsy are CNS depressants, and therefore the potential for additive effects needs to be managed.

Down syndrome

Down syndrome (trisomy 21) is a chromosomal disorder associated with the individual having an extra copy of chromosome 21. However, the impacts of this are widespread, with retarded physical and mental development, a high risk of congenital heart defects, and increased risks of respiratory infections, asthma, epilepsy and leukaemia.

The characteristic craniofacial development in Down syndrome impacts upon the oral cavity. The oral cavity itself is relatively small, and as a result the tongue becomes relatively large (macroglossia). There is an increased incidence of malocclusion, poor food debris clearance, severe xerostomia, and a tendency to mouth breathing, all of which can impact upon oral health. Normal development and eruption of the dentition is also affected, and microdontia is common.

Perhaps surprisingly, studies indicate that the level of caries in Down syndrome may be low, perhaps as a result of increased interdental spacing due to microdontia. However, good preventive care is still important, and oral hygiene training should be provided for both the patient and their carer. While the incidence of caries is relatively low, periodontal disease is prevalent. The increased risk of periodontal disease does not appear to reflect poor oral hygiene, but rather altered immune and inflammatory responses.

As with all patients, good communication skills are the cornerstone to developing an effective and respectful professional relationship with these patients, and engaging with their carers to encourage good oral health.

CHAPTER 16
Endocrine disorders 1

Alan Nimmo

Key Topics

- Introduction to endocrine disorders
- Pituitary disorders, growth hormone and acromegaly
- Thyroid disorders, their impact on oral health and patient management
- Corticosteroids – their role in the stress response, as well as modulating immune and inflammatory responses
- Pregnancy and dental care

Learning Objectives

- Be aware that dental clinicians may be well placed to detect undiagnosed endocrine conditions, such as acromegaly
- Be aware of the impact of thyroid disorders on oral health, and potential issues, such as a thyroid storm
- Be aware that reduced corticosteroid levels may impact upon a patient's ability to cope with stress, whilst chronic, high levels may lead to immune suppression
- Be aware that routine dental therapy is not only safe during pregnancy, but may improve health outcomes for both mother and newborn
- Be aware that declining levels of oestrogen and progesterone associated with the menopause may have a negative impact upon oral health

Essential Dental Therapeutics, First Edition. Edited by David Wray.
© 2018 John Wiley & Sons Ltd. Published 2018 by John Wiley & Sons Ltd.
Companion Website: www.wiley.com/go/wray/dental-therapeutics

Introduction

The endocrine system works together with the nervous system to control many aspects of body function. As a generalization, the endocrine system is responsible for more widespread, longer-term control within our body. However, there is significant communication and coordination between the nervous and endocrine systems, particularly through the hypothalamic-pituitary axis. The pituitary gland itself is commonly viewed as the 'master' gland of the endocrine system, since its endocrine secretions not only have direct influences in the body, but also regulate the activity of other endocrine glands. However, much of the secretory activity of the pituitary gland is controlled by the hypothalamus.

In terms of both dental and medical practice, the endocrine disorder that has the most significant and widespread impact is diabetes mellitus. Because of its significant implications on oral health and the management of patients within the dental clinic, we shall discus diabetes mellitus in a separate chapter. In this chapter we will examine the other endocrine conditions, and the clinical use of exogenous hormones, that may impact upon oral health and the management of dental patients.

Disorders of endocrine function, as well as the use of exogenous hormones, can have widespread impacts on the body, and may affect:

- Growth and development
- Energy metabolism
- Muscle and adipose tissue distribution
- Sexual development
- Fluid and electrolyte balance
- Inflammation and immune responses.

Obviously, a number of these factors may impact upon oral health and patient wellbeing. Endocrine disturbances are normally associated with either hypo- or hyperfunction of the endocrine glands. Disorders may be directly associated with a defect in the endocrine gland responsible for producing a particular hormone (primary disorder). Conversely, a particular endocrine gland may be fully functional, but its' activity may be affected by defective levels of a particular stimulating hormone or releasing factor. This is referred to as a secondary disorder, and is commonly associated with altered

pituitary function. Finally, hypothalamic dysfunction may impact upon pituitary gland function, giving rise to a tertiary disorder.

In terms of this chapter, we will focus on the endocrine disorders, or hormones that may impact upon the dental patient and their oral health.

Pituitary gland

The pituitary gland releases eight major hormones. Six of these, growth hormone, adrenocorticotropin, thyroid-stimulating hormone, prolactin, follicle-stimulating hormone and luteinizing hormone are released by the anterior pituitary, and two, antidiuretic hormone (or vasopressin) and oxytocin, are released by the posterior pituitary. For those hormones that influence the activity of other endocrine glands, we will consider their impacts on oral health separately. In terms of those hormones with direct actions, oral health implications are observed with altered levels of growth hormone, and potentially antidiuretic hormone.

Growth hormone, as the name suggests is important for normal growth and development, but it also has impacts on metabolism, promoting lean body mass and the use of fatty acids as an energy source. In children, the effects of a deficiency in growth hormone, or its activity, will impact upon normal development, and may lead to short stature (pituitary dwarfism). There are impacts in the oral cavity, particularly with mandibular, but also maxillary growth. Normal development of the roots and supporting structures of the teeth is retarded, and malocclusion may be associated with the smaller dental arches. There are also delays in both the normal eruption and shedding of teeth. In adults, the impacts of growth hormone deficiency are more associated with metabolic disturbances, although reduced bone mineral density may be observed. In both children and adults, management is primarily associated with growth hormone replacement therapy, although for children with defective growth hormone receptors, the developmental issues can be managed with the use of insulin-like growth factor 1.

There are also problems associated with excessive growth hormone production. In children, an excess of growth hormone can lead to gigantism associated with increased linear bone growth. Oral and dental development is normally in proportion to the body overall. There is a somewhat different picture associated with growth hormone excess that occurs during the adult years, giving rise to a condition known as acromegaly. Most commonly the condition occurs as a result of neoplasia of the growth hormone secreting cells in the pituitary. After the epiphyseal plates fuse, there can be no increase in stature. Instead, the condition is characterized by disproportionate growth mainly affecting the face, extremities such as the hands, and internal organs. The craniofacial changes tend to be characteristic of the disease, and the onset may be insidious. As such, dental professionals may be best placed to detect some of the early changes. Some of the more obvious oral signs include mandibular prognathism and thickening, increased thickening and height of the alveolar process, the spacing and flaring of anterior teeth, associated malocclusion, and an enlarged tongue. The metabolic implications of growth hormone excess may lead to diabetes mellitus. Management may involve drugs that inhibit growth hormone release, such as the dopamine agonist, bromocriptine, or the somatostatin analogue, octeotide. Stereotactic radiosurgery may also be an option.

Antidiuretic hormone (ADH), or vasopressin, plays an important role in regulating water balance in the body, facilitating the production of a concentrated urine by the kidneys by increasing the water permeability of the collecting ducts, promoting water reabsorption. A deficiency in ADH secretion, or action, leads to a condition known as diabetes insipidus. Like diabetes mellitus, polyuria is a key symptom, but in this case it is associated with the production of large volumes of a dilute urine. These effects may be exacerbated by some medications, such as NSAIDs, which reduce vasopressin's effects. The potential for xerostomia is likely to be the main oral issue. Therapeutic management may involve the vasopressin analogue, desmopressin.

Thyroid gland

Disorders of the thyroid gland are the second most common form of endocrine disease after diabetes mellitus, and a number of these disorders have an autoimmune basis. The thyroid gland plays a very important role in regulating metabolism, but also influences normal growth and development, including tooth eruption. There are three key hormones produced by the thyroid gland, thyroxin (T4) and tri-iodothyronine (T3), commonly referred to as the thyroid hormones, and also calcitonin. The production of T4 and T3 is regulated by the pituitary hormone, thyroid-stimulating hormone (TSH).

Hyperthyroidism

Hyperthyroidism, or thyrotoxicosis, is associated with excessive thyroid hormone secretion leading to a high metabolic rate, and a variety of associated symptoms, including increased skin temperature and sweating, weight loss, nervousness and tachycardia. Patients with hyperthyroidism are prone to cardiovascular disease, including arrhythmias, due to the effects of the hormone on the heart. The two common forms of hyperthyroidism are toxic nodular goitre and diffuse toxic goitre (Grave's disease). Toxic nodular goitre is associated with benign neoplasia, while diffuse toxic goitre has an autoimmune basis, with autoantibodies activating the TSH receptors. This condition is also associated with an increased sensitivity to catecholamines, and the problem of exophthalmos, caused by excessive connective tissue deposition in the orbits.

Hyperthyroidism can be treated surgically, but is more commonly managed by drugs that reduce thyroid hormone production, although these do not address the underlying autoimmune problem. Radioactive iodine (^{131}I) can exert very selective cytotoxic effects on the thyroid follicle cells, while thioureylenes, such as carbimazole, will decrease thyroid hormone synthesis. Beta-adrenergic antagonists may be used for symptomatic control of the problems such as tachycardia and muscle tremors. Corticosteroids, such as prednisolone have been used to manage the exophthalmos, although there is currently an interest in using other disease-modifying immunosuppressant drugs.

In terms of the dental implications, patients with hyperthyroidism are more susceptible to caries and periodontal disease, and may be prone to other oral problems, such as burning mouth syndrome. For patients with existing hyperthyroidism, it is important to assess how well controlled their condition is, and to defer treatment, particularly invasive treatment, in cases of poor disease control. In such situations, it is appropriate to confer with the patient's physician. By the same token, it is important for the dental professional to be able to detect the signs of undiagnosed hyperthyroidism. Patients with hyperthyroidism may exhibit high levels of thyroid or sympathetic activity, with signs of tachycardia, muscle tremors, heightened anxiety and irritability.

The stress associated with dental visits has the potential to exacerbate any cardiovascular issues associated with hyperthyoidism, or potentially precipitate a thyroid storm. As such, these patients may benefit from sedation within the dental clinic. These patients are also likely to be very sensitive to adrenaline-containing products, including local anaesthetic preparations and gingival retraction cords. Such preparations need to be used with caution, particularly on patients who are also being prescribed non-selective beta-blockers for their hyperthyroidism. In this situation, adrenaline will only exhibit vasoconstrictor effects. In terms of analgesia, NSAIDs should be used with caution, as they have the potential to increase the free, circulating levels of thyroxine, increasing the risk of thyrotoxicosis. However, the biggest single concern in terms of managing patients with poorly controlled hyperthyroidism is the potential for a thyroid storm, or thyrotoxic crisis. It is associated with an excessive release of thyroid hormones, and has the potential to be a life-threatening medical emergency.

Hypothyroidism

Hypothyroidism relates to a reduced secretion of thyroid hormones. It may be associated with a loss of thyroid function (primary), or reduced stimulation of the thyroid gland (secondary). There are a number of causes of primary thyroid deficiency, including autoimmune-mediated chronic thyroiditis (Hashimoto's disease) and drug-induced (litium, amiodarone). Diet may also play a role, since a diet that is low in iodine or protein may lead to reduced synthesis of thyroid hormones. These problems are more common in developing countries, since many developed countries have iodine supplementation

programs in place. However, the impact of iodine on thyroid function is 'bell-shaped', and excessive iodine levels can lead to a variety of thyroid pathologies, including hypo- and hyperthyroidism, particularly in susceptible individuals.

As mentioned previously, thyroid hormones are essential for normal development. In infancy, hypothyroidism has major developmental impacts, including normal neurological development, leading to the condition of cretinism. In adults many of the signs of hypothyroidism, or myxoedema, relate to the metabolic dysregulation. Sufferers will have a low metabolic rate, will be cold intolerant, may commonly be overweight, have reduced cardiovascular and respiratory function, anaemia, hypercholesterolaemia, and generalized oedema, with non-pitting skin oedema. Neurological signs may include depression and paraesthesia. There is emerging evidence that thyroid hormone deficiency may play a role in the pathology of epilepsy, through influencing the balance of inhibitory (GABA-ergic) and excitatory (glutaminergic) activity. The medical management of hypothyroidism primarily involves replacement therapy with levothyroxine, with hormone levels being carefully titrated and monitored to prevent hypo- or hyperthyroidism.

Dental patients with hypothyroidism may have enlarged salivary glands, enlarged tongue and glossitis, dysgeusia, delayed dental eruption, and poor periodontal health. In general, patients with managed hypothyroidism should tolerate dental treatment well. However, patients with hypothyroidism are more prone to cardiovascular disorders, so an assessment of cardiovascular health may be the primary consideration prior to dental therapy. In contrast to hyperthyroidism, sedatives, such as benzodiazepines, should be used with caution, since the patients are more susceptible to the sedative effects. However, adrenaline-containing preparations should not be of concern, unless the patient has cardiovascular comorbidity, in which case normal caution should be exercised. Where possible, opioids should be avoided for post-operative analgesia due to patients' increased sensitivity to these agents. Providone-iodine as an antiseptic agent should be used with caution due to the possibility of iodine-induced hypothyroidism.

Parathyroid glands

The parathyroid glands release the peptide hormone, parathyroid hormone which, in adults, is the main hormone controlling blood Ca^{2+} levels. Parathyroid hormone is released when Ca^{2+} levels fall, stimulating osteoclasts to reabsorb bone, and release Ca^{2+} into the blood. Subsequently, as Ca^{2+} levels rise, the stimulus for parathyroid hormone release declines. Another hormone, calcitonin, released from the thyroid gland is also involved in regulating Ca^{2+} ion levels. Calcitonin is secreted when blood Ca^{2+} levels rise, inhibiting bone reabsorption and promoting the deposition of calcium salts in bone matrix. However, while calcitonin is effective in reducing blood Ca^{2+} levels in children, its activity in adults is negligible. It appears to have a greater role during early bone development, but by adulthood, its effects are negligible, and parathyroid hormone dominates in terms of calcium homeostasis.

Primary hyperparathyroidism, is mainly associated with neoplasia of the parathyroid gland, while the secondary condition may be associated with other conditions that lead to hypocalcaemia. The signs of primary hyperparathyroidism are bone lesions associated with excessive osteoclast activity, combined with the impacts of hypercalcaemia. These include the presence of calcium stones in the urinary tract, calcium deposition in soft tissues, gastrointestinal disturbances, and neurologic and neuromuscular disorders. One of the first oral signs is malocclusion due to tooth mobility associated with bone remodelling. However, there may also be defects associated with dental development and eruption. In general, these patients do not require any special management, other than an awareness of the potential risk of bone fracture.

Hypoparathyroidism may be hereditary in origin, or may be acquired as a result of surgical trauma or autoimmune destruction. Because osteoclast activity is low, bones are not significantly affected. Instead the associated hypocalcaemia impacts more on nerve and muscle function. There may be a range of neurological symptoms, and tetany may occur, with the muscles of the larynx being particularly susceptible. Treatment may involve substitution therapy with hydroxycholecalciferol or vitamin D.

In terms of dental management, it is appropriate to request an analysis of serum calcium levels in order to assess the risk of hypocalcaemia-induced arrhythmias and seizures. These patients are more prone to caries, and dental management should be targeted at caries prevention. If hypothyroidism develops during odontogenesis, there may be enamel hypoplasia or failed eruption, while persistent oral candidiasis in a young patient may be a sign of onset of autoimmune polyglandular syndrome.

Adrenal glands

The adrenal glands are a vital element of the endocrine system, and produce a diverse range of endocrine secretions. There are distinct regions within the adrenal gland responsible for the diverse endocrine secretions. The adrenal gland consists of an inner portion, referred to as the adrenal medulla, and an outer, adrenal cortex. The adrenal medulla releases catecholamines, primarily adrenaline, but also noradrenaline and dopamine, into the circulation as part of the systemic sympathetic ('fight-or-flight') response. In addition, the adrenal medulla also secretes progesterone, which we will consider in the next section.

The adrenal cortex is responsible for the production of a number of steroid hormones. The outer, glomerular layer of the cortex is responsible for the production of mineralocorticoids, in particular aldosterone, which regulates salt and water balance through its action on the kidneys, and in turn influences blood pressure. The innermost layer of the cortex is responsible for androgen hormone precursors. The middle layer of the cortex (fascicular or intermediate layer) is responsible for the production of the glucocorticoid hormones, particularly hydrocortisone (cortisol). The glucocorticoids are central to maintaining homeostasis during periods of stress. The glucocorticoids have a variety of metabolic effects, including stimulating hepatic glucose production, mobilizing fatty acids and promoting their metabolism, and breaking down body proteins to use the amino acids for gluconeogenesis. They are also involved in emotional behaviour, have immune suppressant and anti-inflammatory effects, and may slow wound healing and bone deposition. The production and secretion of corticosteroid hormones is primarily under the control of the pituitary hormone, adrenocorticotropic hormone (ACTH).

Addison's disease

Addison's disease is associated with primary adrenal cortical insufficiency. It is relatively rare, being most commonly caused by autoimmune destruction, but can also be caused by infection (particularly TB), trauma, cancer, and haemorrhage associated with anti-coagulant therapy. Glucocorticoid deficiency leads to poor stress tolerance, hypoglycaemia, lethargy, weakness, nausea and vomiting, anorexia and weight loss, while loss of mineralocorticoid function results in dehydration, low blood pressure and fatigue. Decreased adrenal function is coupled to high ACTH levels which leads to hyperpigmentation of the skin as a result of ACTH being very similar to melanocyte-stimulating hormone. These effects will also be observed in the oral cavity, with the gums and oral mucous membranes developing a bluish-black colouration. Treatment of Addison's disease relies on life-long hormone replacement therapy.

One of the key issues associated with long-term (>14 days) corticosteroid therapy is the potential for suppressed adrenal function, and this needs to be taken into account in relation to dental therapy. As mentioned, normal adrenocortical function enables the body to manage stress situations, and that will include dental therapy. In situations where adrenal function is depressed, there is a requirement for supplemental corticosteroid administration for prolonged or stressful dental procedures, which normally represents doubling the patient's normal dose. A subsequent, supplemental dose may also be required on the day following treatment if there is likely to be significant post-operative pain. Adrenal suppression is a function of both the duration of therapy, and the dose used. For patients on low doses (<30 mg hydrocortisone/day) of corticosteroid therapy, there may be no marked suppression. Alternatively, patients on high-dose therapy (>40 mg hydrocortisone/day) may have sufficient corticosteroid levels to enable the body to cope with the clinical stress. In both cases, supplemental treatment may not be required. As such, supplemental corticosteroid is primarily required for patients on long-term moderate dose (30 mg–40 mg hydrocortisone/day) therapy. Supplemental dosing is not required for patients using inhaled or topical corticosteroid therapies. Other strategies for the management of these patients should include morning appointments, managing stress and anxiety, and good local anaesthesia and post-operative analgesia. These strategies can help reduce the risk of an Addisonian crisis, which is a rare, but serious, medical emergency related to insufficient corticosteroid levels.

Cushing's syndrome

Cushing's syndrome, or hyperadrenocorticism, as a condition in itself, is associated with excessive glucocorticoid hormone release, normally associated with neoplasia. The condition may be associated with an adrenal tumour, or as a result of a pituitary tumour, causing excessive ACTH production. The signs of Cushing's syndrome are basically due to the exaggerated actions of cortisol. However, the same syndrome is also observed in patients who are being prescribed prolonged, systemic corticosteroid therapy (iatrogenic Cushing's syndrome). This is not seen in patients who are receiving corticosteroids as a replacement therapy (Addison's disease), but rather when they are being prescribed for their anti-inflammatory and immune suppressive effects (e.g. management of autoimmune disorders or transplant recipients). In terms of the therapeutic management of non-iatrogenic Cushing's syndrome, there is the potential to reduce the synthesis of glucocorticoids. Drugs with an inhibitory action on glucocorticoid synthesis include metyrapone, mitotane and the anti-fungal agent, ketoconazole.

There is a broad range of symptoms associated with Cushing's syndrome, and many relate to the metabolic effects of corticosteroids. Altered fat metabolism leads to an abnormal fat distribution, with a protruding abdomen, subclavicular and cervical fat pads, and rounding and puffiness of the face (moon face). There is also muscle weakness and thinning of the extremities as a result of protein breakdown and muscle wasting. The skin of the arms and legs becomes thin, and bruises easily, and osteoporosis may develop as a result of calcium reabsorption. Deranged glucose metabolism is common, leading to hyperglycaemia and a potential for the development of diabetes. The action of glucocorticoids on the kidneys may lead to excessive potassium loss and hypokalaemia, as well as sodium retention, and resultant hypertension. There is increased gastric acid secretion, which increases the risk of gastric ulceration. The glucocorticoids also may lead to emotional and sleep disturbances, which may appear as depressive-like symptoms.

In terms of the management of patients in the dental clinic, one of the main considerations is the problem of immune suppression and the increased susceptibility to infection. Opportunistic infections, including oral candidiasis may be an issue, and prevention of infections is important. Many patients with asthma may be using inhaled corticosteroids, and while this will not cause systemic immune suppression, deposition of inhaled steroid within the oral cavity may predispose individuals, particularly those with poor inhaler technique. Other issues that need to be managed are the problems of hypertension, hyperglycaemia, depression and impaired wound healing. Finally, corticosteroid use may lead to adrenal suppression, and therefore the need for supplemental corticosteroid doses needs to be examined.

Glucocorticoids represent very powerful anti-inflammatory agents, although their usefulness is limited by their significant side effects. Many of these issues can be circumvented with topical preparations. Corticosteroids, particularly topical preparations, have a wide range of applications in dentistry, including oral surgery. The use of corticosteroids during and after third molar removal and other dentoalveolar surgery, can reduce post-surgical pain, oedema, and help prevent post-operative lingual and inferior alveolar nerve hypersensitivity.

Reproductive hormones

Normal sexual development and reproduction is under the control of a number of hormones, including the female (oestrogen and progesterone) and male (testosterone) sex steroids, the pituitary hormones, follicle-stimulating hormone and luteinizing hormone, and the hypothalamic releasing factor, gonadotrophin-releasing hormone. While these hormones play a role in development, the biggest influence on oral health is seen with oestrogen and progesterone, and in particular the changes in the levels of these hormones during pregnancy, the menopause, and the use of the contraceptive pill. Oestrogen may increase vascularization in the oral mucosa, while decreasing keratinization. Progesterone also acts on the gingival vasculature, causing dilation and increased vascular permeability, which may result in oedema and the infiltration of inflammatory cells. It too may cause vascular proliferation and altered collagen synthesis. Together these factors increase the risk of gingival bleeding and periodontal disease.

Pregnancy

The hormonal changes associated with pregnancy may have negative effects on oral health, and as such good oral care can deliver the best health outcomes for both the mother and developing foetus. However, ironically, pregnancy is also a time when some women may neglect dental visits because of concerns about adverse pregnancy outcomes. However, these concerns are unfounded. Routine preventive, diagnostic and clinical care does not result in adverse outcomes, and is likely to be of benefit to mother and child.

In terms of the direct hormonal influences on oral health, one of the major problems is periodontal disease. As many as 75% of women may develop pregnancy gingivitis, showing signs of gingival oedema, erythema and bleeding. These changes may begin early in pregnancy, and persist before resolving following parturition. While the gingival changes associated with pregnancy gingivitis are no different from other forms of gingivitis, it is caused by the pro-inflammatory effects of oestrogen and progesterone enhancing the inflammatory response. The mucosal changes associated with these hormones may also change the microbial flora in subgingival plaque, increasing the percentage of anaerobic bacteria. Pregnancy can also cause the formation of tumour-like growths in the gingiva, referred to as pregnancy granulomas (epulis gravidarum). This painless lesion develops in areas that are inflamed and irritated, and will normally regress following parturition.

There is an increased risk of caries during pregnancy. Much of this may be due to dietary changes, with increased carbohydrate intake associated with food cravings, and a tendency to regular snacking. There may also be a decline in oral hygiene practices due to concerns about bleeding gums, an enhanced 'gag reflex', and general tiredness. In addition, acid erosion may be associated with the problem of morning sickness, which affects almost 75% of women, particularly during early pregnancy. The hormonal changes may also increase the risk of xerostomia.

Standard dental treatment is not only safe, but is advisable, throughout pregnancy. However, appointments between Weeks 14 and 20 of pregnancy may represent the most comfortable time for patients to undergo therapy since much of the early pregnancy nausea may have resolved by this time, while there are less likely to be significant postural issues associated with the developing foetus. Particularly in later pregnancy, it is important to be careful with patient positioning in the dental chair in order to prevent hypotension. As with the use of all medications during pregnancy, caution should be exercised with dental medications, particularly during the first trimester. There is more safety information associated with established medications. In terms of local anaesthetics lignocaine with adrenaline, and mepivacaine have good safety records. In terms of antibiotic therapy there are a number of antibiotics (e.g. amoxicillin) and antifungals (e.g. nystatin) that may be used. In terms of analgesics, paracetamol is preferred, although codeine is also an option. NSAIDs like ibuprofen are best avoided in the first and third trimesters. In terms of sedation, benzodiazepines should be avoided, but if sedation is essential nitrous oxide may be used in consultation with the patient's medical practitioner.

Contraceptive pill

Oral contraceptives first became available in the 1960s, and these first pills contained relatively high doses of oestrogens and progestogen. It soon became clear that there were potential health risks associated with the early forms of oral contraception, and this lead to the development of the current forms of the contraceptive pill. The two main current forms are the combined pill, with relatively low doses of oestrogen and progestogen, and the progestogen-only pill. These pills produce their effect primarily through interfering with the normal feedback mechanisms that control FSH and LH secretion. There is a common conception that the contraceptive pill may impact upon periodontal health, and much of this view probably arose from the early, high-dose preparations, where the oestrogen and progesterone may have exerted pro-inflammatory effects. As such, the contraceptive pill has been included on the list of medications that influence gingival disease. However, there is a growing view that the current low-dose preparations may not, in themselves, have an impact on periodontal health.

Menopause

The declining levels of oestrogen and progesterone associated with the menopause may also have an impact on oral health. With aging and the menopause, there is a thinning of the oral mucosa, decreased salivary gland function, with associated xerostomia and an increased risk of burning mouth syndrome. Following the menopause, the periodontium becomes more prone to inflammation, with an increase in the prevalence and severity of periodontal disease. The menopause may also lead to increased osteoclast activity. Naturally, oestrogens inhibit osteoclastic activity by promoting the apoptosis of osteoclasts. However, with falling oestrogen levels bone reabsorption starts to outpace bone deposition. This process can underpin the development of osteoporosis, but may also exacerbate alveolar bone reabsorption. The potential use of hormone replacement therapy (HRT) to manage oral symptoms of the menopause is controversial, and not all postmenopausal women appear to benefit from its effects. It has been suggested that short-term HRT could be used to manage persistent oral symptoms, but this needs to be balanced against other health risks, such as reproductive cancers. In general, good oral hygiene practices should represent the mainstay for postmenopausal oral health.

CHAPTER 17

Endocrine disorders 2 – diabetes mellitus

Alan Nimmo

Key Topics

- Introduction to diabetes mellitus
- Type 1 and Type 2 diabetes mellitus
- Systemic and oral signs and symptoms of diabetes
- Diabetes, inflammation and periodontal disease
- Management of diabetes mellius
- Management of the diabetic patient in the dental clinic

Learning Objectives

- Be aware that diabetes mellitus is a condition associated with an absolute or relative deficiency of insulin activity
- Be aware that diabetes mellitus is not a single condition, and that type 2 diabetes, the more prevalent form, is primarily a "lifestyle" disease
- Be familiar with the oral signs of diabetes mellitus, as there is significant potential for dental practitioners to pick up undiagnosed type 2 diabetes
- Be familiar with the link between diabetes (both type 1 and 2) and periodontitis, both in terms of prevalence and severity
- Be aware that patients with diabetes mellitus can significantly benefit from good oral health management
- Be familiar with the strategies that should be used to optimise the treatment of the diabetic patients in the dental clinic

Essential Dental Therapeutics, First Edition. Edited by David Wray.
© 2018 John Wiley & Sons Ltd. Published 2018 by John Wiley & Sons Ltd.
Companion Website: www.wiley.com/go/wray/dental-therapeutics

Introduction

Diabetes mellitus represents the most significant endocrine disorder. In particular, type 2 diabetes is considered the fastest-growing chronic disease, being responsible for approximately 5 million deaths per annum. The term diabetes literally means 'going through' or overflow, and is used to describe conditions where large volumes of urine are excreted. The term mellitus means 'sweet' or 'honey-like', referring to the presence of glucose in the urine. Diabetes mellitus is associated with a lack of secretion or a lack of activity of the hormone insulin, which, in uncontrolled diabetes, results in raised blood glucose levels.

It has been long recognized that there is a link between diabetes mellitus and periodontal disease, and it has been suggested that periodontitis should be considered a formal complication of diabetes. All diabetic patients are at risk of poor oral health and periodontal disease, but the problem is greater in those with poor diabetic control. Importantly, this is a two-way link, with periodontal disease impacting on diabetic control. Because of the impacts of diabetes on oral health, dentists are well placed to pick-up undiagnosed diabetes. Other issues that need to be considered in relation to diabetes mellitus, is that your diabetic patients may be more prone to oral infections. In addition, as a dentist, you have to be able to manage diabetic emergencies, and develop strategies to reduce the risk of such events. The risk of diabetic emergencies is higher in those patients receiving insulin therapy.

Diabetes mellitus

Diabetes mellitus is a condition associated with an absolute or relative deficiency of insulin activity. One of the functions of the hormone insulin is, along with the hormone glucagon, to regulate blood glucose levels. Insulin promotes the uptake of glucose by cells, thereby lowering blood glucose levels. As mentioned, the term diabetes relates to one of the key symptoms, namely polyuria. When uncontrolled, sufferers will produce large volumes of urine, which, unlike normal urine, contains glucose. Normally all of the glucose present in the glomerular filtrate produced by the kidneys is reabsorbed back into the bloodstream. However, if blood glucose levels are too high (>180 mg/ml), the active transport mechanism becomes saturated, and glucose will be lost in the urine. The presence of glucose in the urine has an osmotic effect, drawing water out with it, thereby causing polyuria. Diabetes mellitus should not be confused with diabetes insipidus, where the polyuria is caused by a deficiency of the hormone anti-diuretic hormone (ADH), or vasopressin. As a result of the polyuria, sufferers may also complain of excessive thirst due to dehydration, causing them to drink large amounts of fluid (polydipsia).

Diabetes mellitus is a disorder of insulin availability, but it is not a single disease. Its classification is based around the cause of the problem. The most basic classification of the disorder is indicated by the terms 'type 1' and 'type 2' diabetes. While type 1 diabetes represents what most people envisage as the problem, it accounts for less than 10% of sufferers. The much larger, and steadily growing proportion of sufferers are classified as having type 2 diabetes.

Type 1 diabetes mellitus

Type 1 diabetes is characterized by the destruction of the insulin-producing beta cells in the pancreas, and is divided into two subtypes, type 1A and type 1B. In type 1A diabetes, which was formerly referred to as juvenile-onset diabetes, there is an immune-mediated destruction of the insulin-producing beta cells in the pancreas. This autoimmune reaction results in an absolute lack of insulin, elevated blood glucose levels, and the breakdown of body fats and proteins as an alternative energy source. Type 1B, or idiopathic, diabetes describes cases where there is beta cell destruction, but there is no evidence of an autoimmune reaction. With type 1 diabetes, there is strong evidence for a genetic predisposition involving multiple genes, particularly genes that regulate normal immune responses. The onset of the symptoms of diabetes may occur quite suddenly, normally when the beta-cell mass has been reduced by around 80%. However, type 1 diabetes-associated antibodies may exist for years before the onset of the signs of diabetes. As such, there is a potential for predictive testing, as well as prevention and early control.

The absolute loss of insulin function with type 1 diabetes has marked metabolic effects. In uncontrolled diabetes, a person is unable to transport glucose into fat and muscle cells. As a result, these cells are 'starved' of glucose, and fat and protein breakdown is increased in order to provide an alternative source of energy. Naturally, insulin inhibits lipolysis, while a lack of insulin activates hormone-sensitive lipase. This leads to the release of significant quantities of free fatty acids into the blood stream, and they become the main energy substrate in most tissues. However, low circulating insulin levels combined with high free fatty acid levels leads the liver to produce high levels of acetoacetic acid which cannot be taken and metabolized by peripheral tissues. Some of the acetoacetic acid is converted into acetone and β-hydroxybutyric acid. This combination of chemicals is commonly referred to as ketone bodies, and causes the problem of ketoacidosis. Ketoacidosis is primarily associated with type 1 diabetes. In severe, uncontrolled diabetes, high levels of ketone bodies can cause severe acidosis, which may lead to a diabetic coma and potentially death.

Individuals with type 1 diabetes require insulin-replacement therapy in order to reverse catabolism, control blood glucose levels, and prevent ketoacidosis.

Type 2 diabetes mellitus

Type 2 diabetes is primarily considered a 'lifestyle' disease. Unlike type 1 diabetes, where there is an absolute deficiency of insulin, in type 2 diabetes there is hyperglycaemia associated with a relative insulin deficiency. It is a disorder of both insulin levels (beta cell dysfunction) and insulin function (insulin resistance). Insulin levels may be high, normal or low, but there is insufficient insulin activity to meet the body's needs. In the presence of insulin resistance, insulin cannot function effectively, and hyperglycaemia results. Type 2 diabetes is not associated with autoantibodies. However, with time, and without effective intervention, type 2 diabetes may progress to a stage where insulin-replacement therapy is required.

Lifestyle plays a big role in the development of type 2 diabetes, with approximately 80% of sufferers being overweight. Individuals with upper body obesity (central obesity) are at greater risk. Previously type 2 diabetes was found more in the older population, but it is becoming more common in obese adolescents. It is a progressive condition associated with insulin resistance. That mismatch between insulin supply and demand, initially produces increased beta cell secretion of insulin (hyperinsulinaemia). However, with time, the insulin response declines because of increasing beta cell dysfunction. There are a number of possible reasons for beta cell dysfunction, including cell exhaustion due to chronic stimulation, cell desensitization due to hyperglycaemia, apoptosis of beta cells and cell toxicity caused by increased free fatty acid levels. Initially blood glucose levels are only high after a meal (post-prandial), but eventually fasting levels will also rise. However, most people with type 2 diabetes do not have an absolute insulin deficiency, and therefore are less prone to ketoacidosis.

Insulin resistance not only contributes to hyperglycaemia, but also plays a role in other metabolic abnormalities. These problems include high plasma triglyceride levels, low HDL levels, hypertension, systemic inflammation and vascular disease. These abnormalities are referred to as 'insulin resistance syndrome' or 'metabolic syndrome'.

There are a number of factors that may lead to the development of insulin resistance, and these include both metabolic and inflammatory processes. One hypothesis is that insulin resistance and increased glucose production in obese individuals may stem from increased free fatty acid concentration. Free fatty acids stimulate beta cells to secrete insulin, but chronic and excessive stimulation will cause beta cell failure. They will reduce the sensitivity of the liver to insulin, leading to increased hepatic glucose production, while also causing decreased glucose utilization by peripheral tissues, through inhibiting glucose uptake and glycogen storage. There is also thought to be a link between obesity, inflammation and insulin resistance. Again, hyperlipidaemia is thought to be a key factor. Adipose tissue secretes both pro- and anti-inflammatory mediators, or adipokines. The pro-inflammatory mediators include IL-6 and TNFα. As a result, obesity is associated with a state of chronic, low-grade inflammation. IL-6 has been shown to affect glucose and lipid metabolism by antagonizing the actions of insulin, while TNF-α interferes with lipid metabolism.

Gestational diabetes

Gestational diabetes refers to any degree of glucose intolerance first detected during pregnancy, and most frequently affects women with a family history of diabetes. Timely diagnosis and careful management are essential, since there is a high risk of pregnancy complications, mortality, and fetal abnormality. As such, those considered at significant risk should undergo testing early in pregnancy. Importantly, women with a history of gestational diabetes are at high risk of developing type 2 diabetes 5 to 10 years after delivery.

Other types of diabetes mellitus

Formerly known as secondary diabetes, 'other types of diabetes' describes the development of a diabetic conditions as a result of other conditions and syndromes. Diabetes may occur as a result of pancreatic disease, other endocrine disorders, such as acromegaly and Cushing's syndrome, genetic disorders, exposure to environmental agents including viruses (e.g. mumps) and chemical toxins (e.g. nitrosamines), as well as following treatment with various drugs, including diuretics and antiretroviral therapy.

Signs and symptoms of diabetes

Systemic signs of diabetes

Two of the classic signs of diabetes mellitus, for both type 1 and type 2 diabetics are polyuria, or excessive urination, due to glucose acting as an osmotic diuretic and polydipsia, or excessive thirst, resulting from the associated dehydration. The metabolic imbalances may also result in polyphagia, or excessive hunger, although this is seen more in type 1 diabetics. As a result, weight loss is common with type 1 sufferers, while as a generalization, type 2 sufferers tend to be overweight.

Other general signs may include episodes of blurred vision, due to the osmotic effects of blood glucose on the lens of the eye. Fatigue is a common issue, due to the loss of normal metabolic control. Sufferers may complain of paraesthesia, which is abnormal sensory sensations, commonly referred to as 'pins and needles', caused by damage to peripheral nerves. Diabetics may also be more prone to skin infections. As a generalization, the signs of type 1 diabetes mellitus are likely to appear more rapidly and markedly, while those due to type 2 are likely to develop in a more insidious manner.

The long-term complications of diabetes (both type 1 and 2) occur as a result of the lack of normal metabolic control, and in particular its effects on carbohydrate and lipid metabolism, but also as a result of the chronic low-grade inflammatory response associated with the condition. The common complications associated with diabetes are cardiovascular disease, renal disease, macro- and micro-vascular disorders, diabetic neuropathies and diabetic retinopathy. Along with these, there is an increase in the severity and prevalence of periodontal disease.

Oral signs of diabetes

As dental practitioners, it is important to be aware of the oral signs of diabetes mellitus, as there is significant potential to pick up undiagnosed type 2 diabetes. This may enable earlier medical intervention, and help improve the long-term prognosis for these patients. Obviously, one of the cardinal signs is periodontal disease, with increased rates (approximately 3-fold) and severity, particularly with poorly controlled diabetes. The mechanisms of this are discussed in a separate section. Xerostomia is a common issue, and is presumably associated with polyuria and associated dehydration. The incidence of root caries is increased in diabetics, presumably due to increased root exposure, associated with the progression of periodontitis, combined with poor salivary protection. Diabetic patients are more prone to oral infections, particularly fungal infections with Candida species, presumably as a result of poor salivary flow, high glucose levels, and impaired immune function. The vascular disease associated with diabetes increases the risk of pulp necrosis and periapical abscess development as a result of tissue ischaemia. The vascular and immune

Table 17.1 Systemic and oral signs of diabetes

Systemic signs of diabetes mellitus	Oral signs of diabetes mellitus
Polyuria	Periodontal disease
Polydipsia	Xerostomia
Polyphagia (more likely in type 1)	Root caries
Blurred vision	Oral infections (commonly Candida infections)
Fatigue	Periapical abscesses and pulpal necrosis
Paraesthesia ('pins and needles')	Poor wound healing and risk of post-surgical infection
Skin infections	Increased risk of mucosal conditions (lichen planus, burning mouth syndrome)

dysfunction may also lead to poor wound healing following dental surgery, and an increased risk of post-surgical infections. Diabetic patients may also be more prone to developing oral mucosal disorders, including lichen planus, and burning mouth syndrome. The systemic and oral signs of diabetes are summarized in Table 17.1.

Diabetes, inflammation and periodontal disease

It has been long recognized that there is a link between diabetes and periodontal disease, with both type 1 and type 2 diabetics being equally at risk. There is both an increased prevalence and an increased severity of periodontitis. However, and importantly, periodontal disease also impacts on diabetic control.

The effect of diabetes on periodontal disease has been attributed to the formation of advanced glycation end products (AGEs). AGEs are proteins or lipids that become glycated after exposure to sugars. AGEs are produced as part of normal metabolism, but in diabetes, if blood glucose levels are poorly controlled, the hyperglycaemia causes oxidative stress, and excessive levels of AGEs are formed. These AGEs function as pro-inflammatory mediators in diabetes. AGEs bind to AGE receptors (RAGE) on a variety of target cells, including inflammatory cells. This AGE-RAGE complex activates the key pro-inflammatory transcription factor, nuclear factor kappa B (NF-κB), leading to excessive production of inflammatory mediators, including IL-1, IL-6, TNF-α and PGE2.

In addition, AGEs can accumulate in the basement membrane of blood vessels, and this can impair the migration of leukocytes through the blood vessel wall. Leukocytes can become trapped in the vessel wall, while soluble AGEs can activate the leukocytes leading to immune-mediated vascular damage. This immune-mediated damage is implicated in causing the vascular lesions associated with diabetes. This leukocyte activation also triggers an 'infection-mediated' pathway of pro-inflammatory cytokine up-regulation, further increasing in the destruction of connective tissue.

The inflammatory processes associated with diabetes have a number of significant detrimental effects on periodontal tissues. AGEs themselves have a detrimental effect on the normal, physiological turnover of periodontal tissues, decreasing the renewal of periodontal tissues through an action on collagen molecules. Abnormal neutrophil function, and the antimicrobial chemicals they produce (e.g. lysozyme, HOCl, MMPs), can result in the destruction of healthy tissues. There is evidence to support the concept that neutrophils play a role in the development of periodontitis but, in terms of the tissue damage, neutrophil-induced tissue damage may be more associated with the soft-tissues. The alveolar bone loss associated with periodontitis, is thought to be associated with an imbalance in the RANKL/osteoprotegerin (OPG) ratio. Pro-inflammatory mediators, including IL-1, IL-6 and TNFα stimulate periosteal osteoblasts, altering the expression of a cell-surface protein known as 'receptor activator of nuclear factor-kappa B ligand' (RANKL). Osteoclast precursor cells have a receptor on their surface, the RANK receptor, to which RANKL will bind. The binding of RANKL to osteoclast precursors enhances osteoclast formation and thereby promotes bone reabsorption. Finally, altered immune cell function in diabetes leads to defective local immune responses, and reduced elimination of periodontal pathogens. Uncontrolled diabetes is strongly correlated to increased alveolar bone loss, while good glycaemic control, by reducing AGE production, will help reduce the oral problems.

However, the link between diabetes and periodontitis is a two-way process, and there is evidence that periodontitis may even represent a risk factor for the development of type 2 diabetes. Inflammation directly induces insulin resistance in type 2 diabetic patients, with both IL-1 and IL-6 affecting glucose and lipid metabolism by antagonizing the actions of insulin. There is evidence that periodontal treatment is effective in improving metabolic control and the general health of type 2 diabetic patients.

Diagnosis of diabetes

Diagnosis of diabetes mellitus can be made by performing blood tests. In non-pregnant adults, diagnosis can be based on fasting plasma glucose levels (>7 mmol/L), while in can also be detected with casual plasma glucose tests, where plasma glucose levels are greater than 11.1 mmol/L 2 hours after a meal. However, diabetes is best confirmed by an oral glucose challenge test, by having a patient fast for 8 hours and then drink a solution containing 75g of glucose. Blood glucose levels are measured 2 hours after the glucose challenge, with a blood glucose level above 11.1 mmol/L being indicative of diabetes.

Another valuable test is to measure the levels of glycated haemoglobin (HbA1c). This test gives a long-term picture of blood glucose levels, rather than a snapshot view. The degree of glycation reflects the mean plasma glucose over the life of the red blood cell, and hence reflects blood glucose levels over the previous three months. If the HbA1c concentrations are greater than 48 mmol/mol, this reflects long-term poor glycaemic control, and is associated with diabetic complications, including

microvascular disease. While urine tests for glucose were once the standard approach to diagnosis, they are now largely obsolete. However, urine testing may be useful for detecting and monitoring ketoacidosis, through the presence of ketones in the urine (ketonuria).

Compact blood glucose meters are valuable in terms of enabling diabetic patients to self-monitor their control of their diabetes, but are also essential in the dental clinic to enable the rapid recognition of a hypoglycaemic event in a diabetic patient.

Management of diabetes mellitus

The management of diabetes mellitus differs according to type and severity of the diabetes, and in particular the degree of insulin deficiency, although there are common issues. The desired outcome for both type 1 and type 2 diabetes is to normalize blood glucose levels in order to prevent both short- and long-term complications. Careful management of diet and exercise also play a part in the treatment of both conditions.

The discovery of insulin in 1922 transformed type 1 diabetes from a fatal disease into a manageable condition. As a peptide hormone, it cannot be given orally, and hence is primarily delivered by subcutaneous injection, normally twice daily. The aim with replacement therapy is to keep insulin levels as stable as possible, and hence keep blood glucose levels stable. This is achieved by a variety of possible regimes involving combinations of short-acting and longer-acting insulin analogues, and fast-acting solutions and slower-acting suspensions of insulin. Dietary management is very important since, unlike physiological control, insulin levels do not fluctuate to reflect the body's needs. There has to be an 'artificial' control and matching of insulin and carbohydrate intake. Good dietary routine is essential, and this has to be carefully considered in relation to dental therapy.

The most significant and concerning side effect of insulin is hypoglycaemia. These common events, if severe, can cause permanent brain damage or death. The brain has a very high energy requirement, and is almost totally dependent upon blood glucose as its energy source. While the brain does not need insulin to utilize glucose, it is very sensitive to the effects of hypoglycaemia, and can rapidly progress to energy failure in that situation.

As mentioned, lifestyle is a big factor in the development of type 2 diabetes, providing scope for prevention or decreased severity of the condition. Diet and exercise can reduce the risk of developing diabetes by more than 50%, and can dramatically delay the onset of type 2 diabetes.

In the early stages of type 2 diabetes, effective blood glucose control may be achieved by careful dietary management. However, as the condition progresses, medical management may be required to achieve glucose, lipid and blood pressure targets. Initially oral hypoglycaemic agents may be used to manage blood glucose levels, although eventually approximately one-third of type 2 diabetics will require insulin therapy.

Metformin, a biguanide, is currently the first line oral hypoglycaemic agent. While its mechanism of action is unclear, it is able to reduce gluconeogenesis by the liver, increase glucose uptake and utilization, and reduce blood lipid and cholesterol levels. Metformin does not cause hypoglycaemia, but may cause some gastrointestinal upset.

Another group of oral hypoglycaemic agents are the sulfonylureas, such as tolbutamide and glibenclamide. These agents stimulate pancreatic B cells to secrete insulin by promoting the depolarization of those cells by acting on a specific binding site on ATP-sensitive K^+ ion channels. Sulfonylureas are primarily effective in early type 2 diabetes, as they require sufficient functional B cells to exert their effects. They are generally well tolerated, but have the potential to cause hypoglycaemia. The concerns are greater with longer-acting agents, such as glibenclamide, and less with shorter-acting agents, such as tolbutamide. A number of other medications can increase the risk of hypoglycaemia, and these include non-steroidal anti-inflammatory drugs, warfarin, and some antibacterial agents, including sulphonamides. There are a number of other drugs, including repaglinide and nateglidine, that act at the same binding site on ATP-sensitive K^+ ion channels as the sulfonylureas. While less potent, they have a more rapid and selective action, and are less likely to cause hypoglycaemia.

The glitazones (or thiazolidinediones) are a group of hypoglycaemic agents discovered by chance. The only group member still in clinical use is pioglitazone, while a number of other agents have been withdrawn due to toxicity, especially hepatotoxicity concerns. Pioglitazone enhances the action of endogenous insulin, reducing gluconeogenesis in the liver, and increasing glucose uptake. The hypoglycaemic effects of pioglitazone are additive with other agents, and it may be used in combination with metformin.

Other hypoglycaemic agents include the intestinal α-glucosidase inhibitor, acarbose. It reduces and delays carbohydrate absorption from the gastrointestinal tract, reducing the post-prandial increase in blood glucose. The gliptins (e.g. vildagliptin, linagliptin etc) are synthetic drugs that inhibit the enzyme dipeptidyl peptidase-4, an enzyme associated with normal immune regulation, signal transduction and apoptosis. In addition, it plays a role in glucose metabolism, as it degrades incretins, such as glucagon-like peptide-1 (GLP-1) and gastric inhibitory peptide (GIP). Incretins have a hypoglycaemic action by slowing carbohydrate absorption from the gastrointestinal tract, while also increasing insulin secretion and decreasing glucagon secretion. As a result, inhibition of incretin metabolism enhances their natural actions. There are several agents that mimic the natural action of incretins. Exenatide is a synthetic analogue of an agent in Gila monster venom, which, like the venom, has a hypoglycaemic action, and mimics GLP-1 activity. Liraglutide is a GLP-1 agonist. Both agents increase insulin secretion, decrease glucagon secretion, and slow carbohydrate absorption from the gastrointestinal tract.

Management of the diabetic patient in the dental chair

Patients with diabetes mellitus can significantly benefit from good oral health management, not only in terms of preventing or minimizing the oral health impact of diabetes, but also in terms of improving their overall health. As such, they have a high need for oral health care, with a focus on prevention and early intervention. For diabetics whose condition is well managed, treatment in the primary care setting is appropriate, while those with more severe complications may need to be referred to a hospital setting.

Perhaps one of the most important considerations is the timing of dental appointments. It is essential that appointments do not interfere with the normal meal and medication regimes of the patient. As such, early morning and early afternoon appointments are preferred, since they are less likely to interfere with these routines. In contrast, late morning appointments, where the clinician may be running late are more likely to cause problems. It is also important for patients to be aware that they should not fast before appointments, but should take their food and medications as normal. It is also best to avoid long appointments, and minimize stress within the clinic, as this can cause hyperglycaemia and increase the risk of acidosis.

Diabetic patients, and particularly those on insulin therapy, are more prone to medical emergencies, with a hypoglycaemic episode being of greatest concern in the dental clinic. An accurate, up-to-date medical history is essential, and be aware of recent hypoglycaemic reactions, since these increase the risk of another one. While diabetics are commonly aware of the signs of hypoglycaemia, it is important that dental staff are too, and that they are equipped to deal with an emergency. Oral glucose in the form of gel, tablets or drink are commonly all that is required, although, if the patient becomes unconscious an intramuscular injection of glucagon will be required.

The oral cavity of your patients with diabetes is more susceptible to injury, infection and irritation. Therefore, it is essential to treat infections promptly. However, there is no evidence to support the use of prophylactic antibiotics except in cases where they would be used in the general population. It is also important to remember that surgical procedures which result in oral pain during the post-surgical period may impact on a patient's eating habits, and hence dietary control of their diabetes. As such, appropriate analgesia must be prescribed.

Non-steroidal anti-inflammatory (NSAID) analgesics are best avoided in diabetic patients, in particular if they have impaired renal function as a result of the renovascular complications associated with diabetes. This relates to the physiological role of prostaglandins in regulating renal blood flow, and the tendency for NSAIDs to renal insufficiency in the impaired kidney.

CHAPTER 18

Cardiovascular therapeutics

Roddy McMillan

Key Topics

- Cardiovascular physiology & pathology
- Drugs used in cardiovascular disease
- Cardiovascular medications of relevance to the practice of dentistry

Learning Objectives

- To be able to identify the key components of the cardiovascular system
- To be able to list the main cardiovascular diseases
- To be able to list the different classes of cardiovascular medications
- To be able to identify the medications of relevance to the practice of dentistry and identify the reasons why these medications are of importance to dentistry

Essential Dental Therapeutics, First Edition. Edited by David Wray.
© 2018 John Wiley & Sons Ltd. Published 2018 by John Wiley & Sons Ltd.
Companion Website: www.wiley.com/go/wray/dental-therapeutics

Introduction

Patients with cardiovascular diseases commonly attend for dental treatment. Such patients are often prescribed multiple medications to manage their conditions, several of which have potentially serious implications in the practice of dentistry. Therefore, it follows that dental practitioners should have an up-to-date working knowledge of currently prescribed cardiovascular drugs, coupled with a thorough understanding of how these drugs may impact on the practice of dentistry.

This chapter will briefly consider the important aspects of cardiovascular physiology and pathology before discussing the drugs used in the management of cardiovascular disease. Finally, the effects of cardiovascular medications of relevance to the practice of dentistry will be considered.

Cardiovascular physiology

The cardiovascular system is a collection of organs that function together (organ system), thus permitting blood to circulate and transport: nutrients (such as glucose, amino acids and electrolytes), oxygen, carbon dioxide, hormones and blood cells, to and from the cells of the body. Moreover, the cardiovascular system also: stabilizes temperature and pH, facilitates the body's immune system and maintains homeostasis.

Blood is a fluid consisting of cellular components suspended within a plasma matrix. Blood plasma is the pale yellow liquid component of blood which makes up around 55% of the total blood volume. Plasma comprises mainly of water (up to 95% by volume), in addition to 6–8% dissolved proteins (e.g. serum albumins, globulins, and fibrinogen), glucose, clotting factors, electrolytes (e.g. sodium, calcium, magnesium, chloride and bicarbonate), hormones and carbon dioxide. Plasma plays the role of the chief medium for waste product transportation in the body. The cellular component of blood comprises mainly of red blood cells, white blood cells and platelets.

The main components of the human cardiovascular system (CVS) are the heart, blood and blood vessels. In simple terms, the CVS is considered to be a 'closed' system (blood never leaves the network of arteries, veins and capillaries), which comprises of the pulmonary circulation ('loop' through the lungs allowing oxygenation of the blood) and the systemic circulation ('loop' through the rest of the body to deliver oxygen). The heart pumps oxygenated blood to the body and deoxygenated blood to the lungs (see Figure 18.1). The coronary circulation provides the blood supply to the cardiac muscles – originating near the root of the aorta from two arteries: the right and left coronary arteries. The majority of cardiac perfusion occurs during diastole (relaxation of heart muscle); with blood then returning through the coronary veins into the right atrium.

The circulation allows oxygen and nutrients to diffuse from the blood vessels and enter interstitial fluid, which carries oxygen and nutrients to the target cells, with carbon dioxide and waste products travelling in the opposite direction.

Cardiovascular pathology

Cardiovascular diseases involve the heart or blood vessels and include: ischaemic heart disease (IHD), stroke, hypertension, cardiac arrhythmias, venous thromboembolism and peripheral vascular disease (PVD). Cardiovascular diseases are the leading cause of death globally, and tend to become more prevalent with increasing age. The most common cause of cardiovascular disease is atherosclerosis, which is the occlusion and thickening of the systemic arterial vessels due to a chronic inflammatory response. Predisposing factors for atherosclerosis formation include: tobacco smoking, hypertension, hypercholesterolaemia, excessive alcohol consumption, obesity and diabetes mellitus. Atherosclerosis is the underlying mechanism in IHD, PVD and many strokes.

Hypertension

Hypertension is a chronic condition characterized by raised arterial blood pressure. Blood pressure is expressed as two measurements – the systolic and diastolic pressures. The systolic pressure is the maximum pressure of the arterial system – which occurs during systole (contraction of the cardiac muscles). Conversely, the diastolic pressure is the minimum arterial pressure, which occurs during

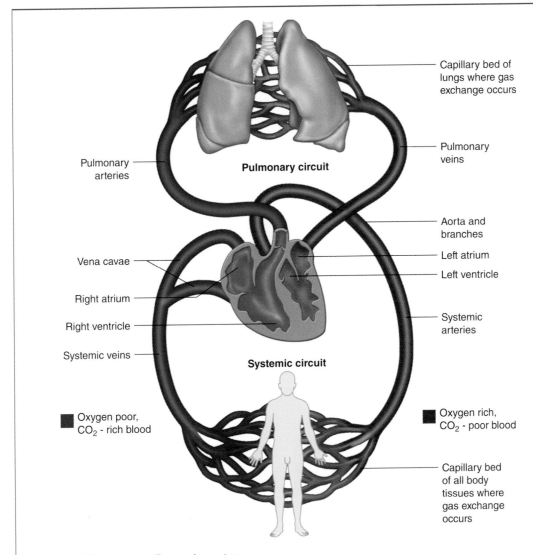

Figure 18.1 The human cardiovascular system.

diastole (relaxation of the cardiac muscles). Blood pressure is represented as the systolic pressure over the diastolic pressure, for example 120/80. Normal blood pressure at rest is within the range of 100–140 millimetres of mercury (mmHg) for systolic and 60–90 mmHg for diastolic. In adults, hypertension is present when blood pressure measured at rest is persistently at or above 140/90 mmHg.

Hypertension is often asymptomatic and is usually identified by the screening of blood pressure by healthcare professionals, or by patients using electronic blood pressure monitors at home. Sustained hypertension over a prolonged period is a major risk factor for hypertensive heart disease (e.g. left ventricular hypertrophy, cardiac failure), coronary artery disease, stroke, aortic aneurysm, chronic kidney disease and peripheral arterial disease.

Hypertension is classified as either essential (primary) hypertension or secondary hypertension. Most cases of hypertension (90–95%) are classed as primary hypertension; defined as high blood pressure with no obvious underlying cause. The remaining 5–10% of cases are considered to be secondary hypertension; hypertension due to an identifiable pathology, for example chronic kidney disease, excess aldosterone production (e.g. Conn's syndrome) or excess catecholamine production (e.g. pheochromocytoma).

Cardiac failure

Cardiac failure occurs when the heart is no longer able to function sufficiently well enough to maintain the blood flow requirements of the body. The common causes of cardiac failure include coronary artery disease, previous myocardial infarction, hypertension and valvular heart disease. Cardiac failure is loosely categorized into left-sided heart failure (reduced ability of left ventricle to send blood to peripheral circulation) and right-sided heart failure (reduced ability to send blood to the lungs). Biventricular failure (i.e. both sides of the heart) is fairly common, and often failure of one side of the heart will lead to failure of the other side.

Cardiac arrhythmia

Cardiac arrhythmias are a group of conditions in which the cardiac rhythm is irregular, too fast, or too slow. Cardiac arrhythmias can be identified by feeling a patient's pulse, or from an electrocardiogram (ECG). In an adult, a cardiac rhythm at rest that is too fast (above 100 beats per minute) is called tachycardia; and a heartbeat that is too slow (below 60 beats per minute) is called a bradycardia. Many arrhythmias are not particularly serious, although some predispose a person to complications such as heart failure, stroke or on occasions cardiac arrest and death.

Venous thromboembolism

Venous thromboembolism comprises of deep vein thrombosis (DVT) and pulmonary embolism. DVT is the formation of a blood clot (thrombus) within a deep vein, predominantly in the legs. Pulmonary embolism, is a potentially life-threatening complication caused by the detachment (embolization) of a thrombus which travels to the lungs and becomes lodged in the pulmonary arterial supply.

The three principle factors which contribute to the development of deep vein thromboses comprise Virchow's triad — venous stasis, hypercoagulability or changes in the endothelial blood vessel lining. Hypercoagulability can be congenital (e.g. Factor V Leiden thrombophilia, Antithrombin III deficiency) or acquired (e.g. anti-phospholipid syndrome, polycythaemia vera).

Peripheral vascular disease

Peripheral vascular disease (PVD), also known as peripheral artery disease, is the pathological occlusion of the arteries that don't supply the brain or the heart. Morbities associated with PVD include: skin ulceration, infection, tissue necrosis or limb amputation. The primary mechanism for narrowing of the peripheral arteries is atherosclerosis – the main risk factor being cigarette smoking, in association with other factors such as diabetes mellitus, hypertension and hypercholesterolaemia. Not surprisingly, PVD is often co-morbid with ischaemic heart disease and stroke, due in large part to the common risk factors shared between the conditions.

Stroke

Stroke, previously known also as cerebrovascular accident (CVA) is characterized by impaired cerebral perfusion, leading to infarction and death of brain tissue. There are primarily two main types of stroke: the most common being ischaemic (due to lack of adequate blood flow), followed by haemorrhagic (due to an intracranial bleed). Hypertension is the most significant risk factor for stroke, followed by other cardiovascular disease risk factors, for example cigarette smoking, hypercholesterolaemia, diabetes mellitus, atrial fibrillation (cardiac arrhythmia) and anticoagulant medications. The morbidity of stroke is very variable and can range from negligible permanent neurological deficit to permanent muscle weakness, paralysis and death.

Drugs used in cardiovascular disease

The Drugs used in cardiovascular disease will now be discussed in turn. These are listed in Table 18.1.

Table 18.1 Drugs used in the management of cardiovascular disease

Anticoagulants
Angiotensin-converting enzyme inhibitors
Angiotensin II receptor blockers
Beta blockers
Calcium channel blockers
Diuretics
Statins
Vasodilators
Antiarrythmics

Anticoagulants

Anticoagulants are medications that aim to prevent the coagulation (clotting) of blood and are primarily used to prevent thrombotic disorders, for example stroke, myocardial infarction, DVT, pulmonary embolus. These drugs are considered in detail in Chapter 18.

Angiotensin-converting enzyme inhibitors

The angiotensin-converting-enzyme inhibitor (ACEi) is an oral medication used principally for the treatment of hypertension and congestive heart failure. The most commonly prescribed ACEis include: captopril, enalapril, lisinopril, perindopril and ramipril.

The pharmacodynamics of ACEis involve the blocking of angiotensin converting enzyme (ACE) which antagonizes angiotensin I conversion to angiotensin II – which are integral components of the renin-angiotensin-aldosterone system (Figure 18.2). Therefore, ACEis lower arteriolar resistance and increase venous capacity, decrease circulating blood volume and increase natriuresis (urinary excretion of sodium) – leading to lowering of blood pressure and a decreased work load on the heart.

The indications of ACEis are numerous, and include: hypertension, congestive cardiac failure, diabetic nephropathy and the long-term management of myocardial infarction.

ACEis are to be used with caution in patients with renal impairment – they can occasionally cause impairment of renal function and hyperkalaemia. Concomitant ACEi treatment with NSAIDs increases the risk of renal damage – hence NSAIDs should be used with caution in such patients.

Although generally well tolerated, ACEis do produce adverse effects, which include: a troublesome cough (related to accumulation of substances normally metabolized by ACE e.g. bradykinin or tachykinins), profound hypotension, renal impairment and occasionally angioedema.

Angiotensin II receptor blockers

The Angiotensin II receptor blockers (ARBs) are a group of orally administered antihypertensive AT_1-receptor antagonists – such that they modify the renin-angiotensin-aldosterone system by blocking the activation of angiotensin II AT_1 receptors (Figure 18.2). Blockage of AT_1 receptors results in vasodilation, reduced secretion of vasopressin, and reduces production of aldosterone, which combine to reduce blood pressure. Examples of ARBs include: azilsartan, candesartan, eprosartan, irbesartan, losartan, olmesartan, telmisartan, and valsartan. The ARBs have similar pharmacodynamics properties to ACEis; however, unlike ACE inhibitors, ARBs don't inhibit the breakdown of kinins, therefore are less likely to cause the persistent dry cough which can complicate ACEi therapy. They are therefore a useful alternative for patients who have to discontinue an ACEi because of persistent cough.

Side-effects of ARBs are usually relatively mild, and include: hypotension, hyperkalaemia and occasionally angioedema. In a similar fashion to ACEi therapy, ARBs should be used with caution in patients with renal impairment.

Beta blockers

Beta-adrenoceptor blocking agents, better known as beta blockers, block the beta-adrenoceptors found in the heart, bronchi, peripheral vasculature, pancreas and liver. Stimulation of the β1 receptors by adrenaline and noradrenaline induces a positive chronotropic (faster heart rate) and inotropic effect (stronger contractions) on the heart, in addition to increasing cardiac conduction velocity. Stimulation

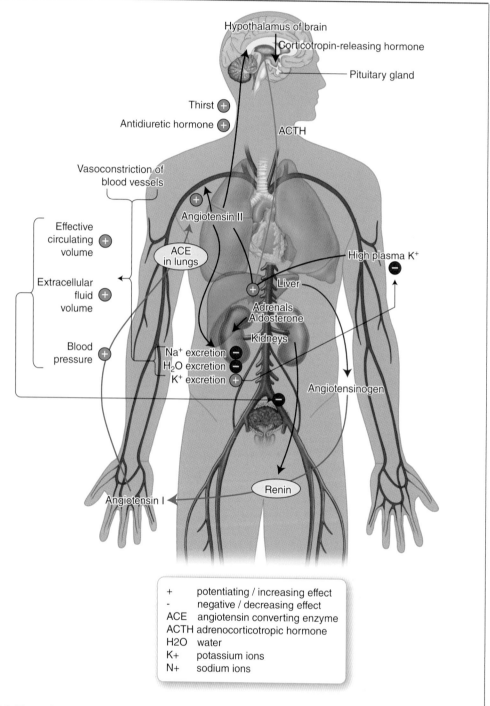

Figure 18.2 The renin-angiotensin-aldosterone system.

of the β1 receptors in the kidney lead to renin release. Stimulation of the β2 receptors results in smooth muscle relaxation, induces skeletal muscle tremor and increases liver and skeletal muscle glycogenolysis. Stimulation of the β3 receptors induces lipolysis. Beta blockers inhibit adrenaline and noradrenaline sympathetic activity – such that they reduce heart rate, force of cardiac contraction, reduce tremor and physical excitement; however, they increase blood vessel dilation and bronchial smooth muscle constriction.

As a result of their pharmacodynamics, beta blockers are used for a variety of cardiovascular diseases, such as: hypertension, arrhythmia, angina, myocardial infarction and heart failure. Moreover, beta blockers are used in other conditions, such as in the management of anxiety, migraine and thyrotoxicosis.

Beta blockers are mostly administered orally, although some such as labetalol and metopralol can be given intravenously. Some beta blockers, for example acebutol, pindolol and oxprenol, demonstrate intrinsic sympathomimetic activity – such that these agents exert mild agonist activity at the beta-adrenergic receptor while simultaneously acting as a receptor site antagonist. Therefore, such drugs can be useful in patients suffering from excessive bradycardia, or coldness of the extremities.

Beta blockers can induce bronchospasm and hence should ideally be avoided in asthmatic patients. In asthmatic patients who require a beta blocker, a more cardioselective (acting mainly on β1 receptors) should be employed, for example atenolol, bisoprolol, metoprolol or nebivolol. Moreover, as beta blockers slow the heart and can depress the myocardium, they are contraindicated in patients with second or third degree heart blocks. In addition, beta blockers can induce nightmares; although the more water soluble beta blockers, for example atenolol, celiprolol, nadolol and sotalol, are less likely to cross the blood-brain barrier, hence are less likely to cause sleep disturbance and nightmares. Beta blockers can induce episodes of hypo or hyperglycaemia in patients with or without a diagnosis of diabetes mellitus – hence cardioselective beta blockers may be preferred in such circumstances.

Calcium channel blockers

Calcium channel blockers are drugs that disrupt the movement of calcium ions through the voltage-dependent calcium channels involved with the contraction of skeletal, smooth, and cardiac muscles, reduction in cardiac electrical activity and the regulation of aldosterone and cortisol secretion in the adrenal cortex. Calcium channel blockers reduce arterial tone, reduce the force of myocardial contraction, reduce heart rate, and reduce aldosterone production – which results in a reduction in blood pressure and cardiac workload. Calcium channel blockers are primarily used as antihypertensives, although are often prescribed for angina and arrhythmias.

The molecular structure of calcium channel blockers vary and as such they vary in their pharmacodynamics and have a greater variation in their therapeutic effects compared to beta blockers. The most commonly prescribed class of calcium channel blocker are the dihydropyridine (DHP) calcium channel blockers (e.g. amlodipine, felodipine and nifedipine); which are principally used as antihypertensives due to their vasodilating properties. The non-DHP calcium channel blockers include the benzothiapines (diltiazem), which possesses antihypertensive and cardiac depressant qualities – making diltiazem useful in angina, arrhythmias and hypertension. Moreover, the phenylalkylamine calcium channel blockers (e.g. verapamil) are relatively selective for the myocardium, and hence are often used to treat angina. Verapamil is often used in the management of supraventricular tachycardia, due to its antiarrhythmic properties.

The side-effects of calcium channel blockers are variable, although common to most are the adverse-effects associated with vasodilation such as flushing, headache and ankle swelling.

Diuretics

Diuretic medications are primarily used to treat hypertension, heart failure and liver cirrhosis. There are several different classes of diuretic, each with different pharmacodynamics and indications.

Loop diuretics:

'Loop diuretics' such as furosemide, are potent diuretics which act by inhibiting the kidney's reabsorption of sodium and chloride by acting upon the ion transporters in the nephron's loop of Henle resulting in increased urine production, decreased renal blood flow and reduced circulating volume. Loop diuretics are mainly used to treat oedema in heart failure and treatment-resistant hypertension.

Thiazide diuretics:

Thiazide diuretics (e.g. bendroflumethiazide, chlortalidone, indapamide and metolazone), are moderately potent diuretics that inhibit sodium reabsorption at the beginning of the nephron's distal convoluted tubule – leading to increased urine production and reduced circulating volume. In addition to the management of heart failure, low dose thiazides are frequently used in hypertension, as they can produce an optimal blood pressure lowering effect with minimal electrolyte disturbance.

Potassium sparing diuretics:

Potassium-sparing diuretics include the weak diuretics amiloride and triamterene, and the aldosterone antagonists, eplerenone and spironolactone. Amiloride and triamterene are weak diuretics which cause potassium retention, hence are given concomitantly with thiazide or loop diuretics when hypokalaemia is an issue. Spironolactone inhibits the effects of the mineralocorticoids, primarily aldosterone, by displacing them from the mineralocorticoid receptors in the cortical collecting duct of the renal nephrons. The net result of spironolactone is a decrease in the reabsorption of sodium and water, while limiting the excretion of potassium. Triamterene directly blocks the epithelial sodium channels on the lumen aspect of the nephron collecting tubule, thus reducing the exit of potassium into the urine.

Carbonic anhydrase inhibitors:

Carbonic anhydrase inhibitors (e.g. acetazolamide and methazolamide) inhibit carbonic anhydrase, an enzyme associated with the nephron's proximal convoluted tubule – the results of which include, bicarbonate accumulation in the urine and decreased sodium absorption.

The side-effects of diuretics are variable, although common to most are gastrointestinal upset and electrolyte disturbance.

Statins

The statins (atorvastatin, fluvastatin, pravastatin, rosuvastatin, and simvastatin) or HMG-CoA reductase inhibitors are a class of drug used to lower cholesterol, one of the key risk factors in the development of cardiovascular disease. The enzyme HMG-CoA reductase is a key component of the liver's metabolic pathway that produces the majority of the body's cholesterol. Statins act by competitively inhibiting HMG-CoA reductase, thus reducing cholesterol production.

It is proposed that in addition to their cholesterol lowering function, statins may act on several different levels to prevent cardiovascular disease – improved endothelial integrity, atheromatous plaque stabilization, inflammatory response modulation and thrombus inhibition.

Statins appear to be effective in preventing heart disease in those with high cholesterol, with no history of heart disease. Statins have also been found to reduce mortality in patients with existing cardiovascular disease.

Statins can be associated with myalgia, myopathy, myositis, rhabdomyolysis and liver impairment – hence should be issued with caution in those at risk of myopathy or liver disease.

Vasodilators

Nitrates (e.g. glyceryl trinitrate, isosorbide mononitrate, isosorbide dinitrate) have a useful role in angina. Nitrates are potent coronary vasodilators; however, their primary clinical benefit derives from a reduction in venous return, which reduces the left ventricular workload.

Once administered nitrates are denitrated to nitric oxide, thus supplementing existing blood concentrations of nitric oxide (also known as endothelium-derived relaxing factor).

The main adverse effects are related to their potent vasodilation properties – headache, flushing and postural hypotension.

Nicorandil is an oral vasodilator used in the treatment of angina, which acts as a potassium channel agonist. The stimulation of the potassium channels leads to an inhibition of voltage gated calcium channels – resulting in reduced smooth muscle tone and coronary artery vasodilation. Nicorandil can cause gastrointestinal upset, flushing, and of note, oral and perianal ulceration.

Antiarrhythmics

Antiarrhythmics drugs are used to manage cardiac arrhythmias, for example atrial fibrillation, atrial flutter, ventricular tachycardia, and ventricular fibrillation. Arrhythmias are loosely divided into supraventricular arrhythmias (a cardiac conduction problem originating at or above the atrioventricular node), and ventricular arrhythmias (originating within the ventricular conduction system). Many of the drugs used in the treatment of abnormal cardiac rhythms have a therapeutic role in a variety of other cardiovascular diseases.

Adenosine is an intravenous drug with a very short half-life, usually the treatment of choice for terminating paroxysmal supraventricular tachycardia.

Dronedarone is an orally administered multichannel blocking antiarrhythmic drug, used as an alternative for the maintenance of sinus rhythm after cardioversion, in patients with paroxysmal or persistent atrial fibrillation.

The calcium channel blocker verapamil is usually effective for supraventricular tachycardia. It is often used as an initial intravenous bolus dose followed by oral therapy.

Digoxin is a cardiac glycoside derived from digitalis, extracted from the foxglove plant. Digoxin is an inotrope (increases the force of myocardial contraction) and reduces conductivity within the atrioventricular node. As a result, digoxin is used to manage atrial fibrillation and atrial flutter; although beta blockers and calcium channel blockers (diltiazem and verapamil) are usually tried initially. Moreover, digoxin is used as a second line treatment for heart failure, in those who have not responded well to 1st line treatment, such as a combination of ACEi with a beta blocker. Although digoxin doesn't improve mortality in heart failure patients,

it improves both the symptoms of heart failure and exercise tolerance.

Drugs used for the management of both supraventricular and ventricular arrhythmias include amiodarone, flecainide, propafenone and beta blockers. Amiodarone may be administered intravenously as well as by mouth, and has the advantage of causing little or no myocardial depression. Flecainide is a sodium channel blocking antiarrhythmic agent, which is used for a variety of supraventricular and ventricular arrhythmias. Propafenone is an oral preparation used both for the prophylaxis and treatment of ventricular arrhythmias, and in some supraventricular arrhythmias. Beta blockers are used in the management of supraventricular and ventricular arrhythmias. Intravenous beta blockers (e.g. propranolol) can be used to achieve rapid control of ventricular rate.

Although no longer a first choice antiarrhythmic, intravenous lidocaine is a sodium channel blocking drug which can be used for the treatment of ventricular tachycardia in the haemodynamically stable.

Efects of cardiovascular medications of relevance to dentistry

It has been suggested that around 15% of patients using cardiovascular medications will have detectable oral adverse-effects. Among the many side-effects, the most common are xerostomia, followed by lichenoid reactions and dysgeusia. It is important that the dental practitioner be aware of the potential for oral manifestations of cardiovascular medications – as it may be that they will be the first to identify any potential problem. It is important to remember that in the case of a suspected adverse drug reaction affecting the mouth, any proposed changes to the patients prescribed medications should be first discussed with the prescribing clinician, for example general medical practitioner or cardiologist.

Xerostomia

Dry mouth symptoms (xerostomia) is a common complaint in the general population (ranges from

10–46%); moreover, xerostomia is recognized as a side-effect of over 500 different prescribed medications. Oral dryness symptoms secondary to cardiovascular medications is by far the most common oral side-effect of these medications, affecting around 7.5% of such patients. Xerostomia in patients taking cardiovascular drugs is more common in those with comorbid diabetes mellitus and females mirroring the trends seen in the general population. Oral dryness is most commonly reported in those taking antihypertensive medications – chiefly beta blockers, diuretics and ACEi.

Oral lichenoid reactions

Oral lichenoid reactions and oral lichen planus possess similar clinical and histological presentations. An oral lichenoid reaction is a chronic inflammatory mucosal disorder, characterized by a T-lymphocyte mediated inflammatory response likely to represent a type IV (cell mediated) hypersensitivity reaction.

Often an oral lichenoid reaction to a given medication can only be confirmed if the lesion appeared following initiation of the drug, resolves following drug cessation, and reoccurs after a re-challenge of the offending medication. An oral lichenoid reaction is reported to occur in around 3% of patients taking cardiovascular medications, the most common culprits amont others being antihypertensives, in particular ACEi and beta blockers, and aspirin.

Taste disturbances

Taste disturbance associated with medications are fairly common and can present with either a reduced sense of taste (hypoguesia), or an altered, and often unpleasant taste sensation (dysgeusia). As a group, ACEi are associated with taste disturbance. In general, medication associated taste disturbances tend to resolve within 2 to 3 months, even when the offending drug is continued.

Oral ulceration

Drug associated oral ulceration secondary to cardiovascular medications can occur. Inappropriate application of aspirin, whereby it is left in prolonged contact with the oral mucosa, will often result in a localized chemical 'burn'. Although, this tends to be a more common occurrence in patients with oral pain such as toothache, care must be taken in vulnerable patients who use aspirin for cardiovascular disease, such as stroke patients who have difficulty in swallowing. Persistent or 'fixed' oral ulceration secondary to cardiovascular drugs are not particularly uncommon in patients using the angina treatment nicorandil which is also linked to the development of perianal drug related ulceration. Moreover, some beta blockers and the ACEi captopril have been associated with oral ulceration. Prompt and complete resolution of the oral ulceration usually follows cessation of the offending drug.

Drug induced pemphigus vulgaris is a rare and potentially fatal, mucocutaneous autoimmune blistering condition which is associated with oral ulceration, the condition has been linked with ACEi treatment.

Drug-related gingival enlargement

Gradual, painless fibrous overgrowth of the gingivae can occur as a result of calcium channel blocker therapy with nifedipine, diltiazem, verapamil and amlodipine being among the most commonly reported causative agents. In the case of calcium channel blockers, the mechanism seems to be related to the blockade of calcium channels on the fibroblasts, leading to interference with the normal fibroblast cell-death mechanisms. It is generally accepted that there is a plaque-associated inflammatory component in drug-induced gingival hyperplasia, as optimization of oral hygiene will commonly lead to regression of the lesions. Cessation of the offending drug will often, but not always lead to resolution of the hyperplasia; hence surgical revision occasionally is employed.

Angioedema

Angioedema of the face and mouth can occur as a result of ACEi use in around 0.1–6% of patients using ACEi. Angioedema is oedematous swelling as a result of increased vascular permeability which, in the case of ACEi associated angioedema, tends to occur mostly in the head and neck region. ACEi induced angioedema is as a result of bradykinin accumulation due to ACE inhibition in susceptible individuals. Some patient with ACEi-induced angioedema may still have recurrent bouts of swelling despite cessation of the drug.

Drug related angioedema may also be linked with NSAIDs such as aspirin – as a result of mast cell membrane destabilization and consequent degranulation and release of histamine and other inflammatory mediators.

Oral burning symptoms

Drug-related oral burning symptoms can rarely be associated with ACEi use, and seem to resolve spontaneously upon cessation of the drug.

Haemorrhage

Abnormal haemorrhage following invasive oral surgical procedures (e.g. extraction, inferior dental nerve block) can occur in patients taking medications that affect platelet function (e.g. aspirin, clopidogrel), and coagulation (e.g. warfarin, dabigatran). It is important, therefore, that the dental surgeon has knowledge about how to conduct treatments safely on such patients, and when it is appropriate to refer the patient to the specialist setting. In patients who are on treatment that may increase the bleeding tendency, it is recommended that local measures to reduce the risk of haemorrhage are employed in all cases, such as placement of a haemostatic absorbable sponge and suturing of the extraction sockets. Ideally, one should avoid prescribing post-operative NSAIDs in patients taking anticoagulants.

It is generally considered safe to conduct minor oral surgery in patients who are taking antiplatelet medications, such as aspirin and clopidogrel, and heparins. In cases of major surgery where blood loss is expected, or re-bleeds may be serious (unlikely to apply to oral surgery), clopidogrel can be discontinued 7 days before elective surgery if the antiplatelet effect is not desirable.

In patients who take warfarin, current practice suggests that the INR should be measured no more than 72 hours before extractions, sub gingival scaling, infiltrations or administration of an inferior dental block. In patients known to have unstable INRs, the INR should be assessed within the 24 hours preceding the treatment. It is considered relatively safe to conduct oral surgical procedures in patients who have an INR score of less than 4.0 prior to surgery. In cases where the INR score is above 4.0, the dental surgeon should, in the first instance, liaise with the anticoagulation service, who could advise on a suitable regime to reduce the INR safely before surgery. Following dental extractions in warfarin patients, the sockets should be packed and sutured in all cases. Currently, it is not possible to measure the level of anticoagulation induced by the direct thrombin inhibitors (e.g. dabigatran) and factor Xa inhibitors (e.g. rivaroxaban). With regards to the oral surgical management of patients taking these novel anticoagulants, the consensus of opinion recommends not to adjust the dose or stop the drugs, but employ local haemostatic measures and avoid post-operative prescription of NSAIDs.

CHAPTER 19

The respiratory system

Martyn Ormond

Key Topics

- Overview of the respiratory system
- Common drugs used in the management of respiratory disorders and their pharmacology
- Implications for dentistry

Learning Objectives

- To describe the pharmacological management of respiratory disorders
- To understand the main drug categories and describe their mechanism of action, indications and adverse effects
- To understand the implications for dentistry

Essential Dental Therapeutics, First Edition. Edited by David Wray.
© 2018 John Wiley & Sons Ltd. Published 2018 by John Wiley & Sons Ltd.
Companion Website: www.wiley.com/go/wray/dental-therapeutics

Introduction

This chapter considers the drugs used to treat respiratory tract diseases and the implications for the dental practitioner. First there is a brief consideration of the physiology of the respiratory tract followed by a consideration of the most prevalent lower respiratory conditions, asthma and chronic obstructive pulmonary disease (COPD). Thereafter is a consideration of other common respiratory tract disorders, rhinitis and cough (see Table 19.1 for the key sections of this chapter). There follows a description of the drugs used to manage respiratory conditions and finally the implications of prescribing these drugs for the practise of dentistry.

Respiratory physiology

The respiratory tract consists of all anatomical structures involved in respiration, from the nose to the alveoli. It is divided into 2 parts: the upper respiratory tract which includes all structures outside the thorax (nose, nasopharynx, pharynx, larynx and trachea) and the lower respiratory tract, which relates to structures within the thorax (ribs and intercostal muscles, trachea, bronchi and great vessels, pleurae and pleural cavities and the lungs).

The respiratory tree is further subdivided. The trachea divides into the right and left bronchi, then bronchioles, respiratory bronchioles, alveolar ducts and finally ends in the alveoli where gaseous exchange occurs. It is lined by respiratory epithelium with both mucus producing Goblet cells and microvilli. Smooth muscle is present at all levels.

The lungs have dual circulation. The bronchial circulation is part of the systemic circulation and supplies the lung parenchyma, airways and pleurae. The pulmonary circulation, from the right side of the heart, allows for exchange of oxygen and carbon dioxide between blood and air.

For gas exchange to occur air must flow in and out of the respiratory system. Ventilation of the lungs ensures air is delivered to the alveoli to allow gas exchange and maintenance of blood gases. The respiratory muscles as well as lung elasticity and airway resistance influence effective ventilation. Many lung diseases affect the physical properties of the lungs impacting on gas exchange. For example, obstructive disorders narrow airways resulting in air trapping, whereas restrictive disorders stiffen the lungs preventing normal expansion. Airway resistance, through increased tone of the smooth muscle lining plays an important role is asthma.

Control of ventilation is complex, involving the brainstem as well as a wide range of receptors including central and peripheral chemoreceptors, arterial receptors, pain receptors and receptors lining the lungs, airway and chest wall. All of these result in coordinated ventilation and responses to physiological conditions.

Asthma

Asthma is the commonest chronic inflammatory disease of the airways resulting in recurrent reversible obstruction to airflow and increased mucus production. It is increasing in both prevalence and severity worldwide. Children are often affected. It is characterized by intermittent episodes of wheezing, shortness of breath, chest tightness and nocturnal cough. Severe attacks can result in life-threatening hypoxaemia.

The symptoms are a result of constriction of bronchial smooth muscle, oedema of the mucosal lining of the small bronchi and plugging of the bronchial lumen by both mucus and inflammatory cells. There is hyper-reactivity of the bronchi to a wide range of stimuli including chemicals, drugs, exercise and cold air. Asthma is often divided into allergic (extrinsic), in which there is sensitization to allergens, and non-allergenic (intrinsic), however there is significant overlap. The pathogenesis of asthma is a combination of both genetic and environmental factors.

Table 19.1 Chapter key sections
Respiratory physiology
Asthma
COPD
Rhinitis
Cough
Drugs used in respiratory disease
Implications for dentistry

Two main phases of asthma attacks have been described: immediate phase and late phase. A number of immune cells and cytokines are involved in both the initiation and potentiation of an attack. These targets form the basis for the prevention and management of asthma.

Asthma suffers have activated T cells, T-helper 2 cells (Th2 cells), in the bronchial mucosa. These release multiple cytokines that are chemotactic to other immune cells, in particular eosinophils. Interleukin 5 (IL-5) and granulocyte-macrophage colony-stimulating factor encourage these eosinophil's to produce cysteinyl leukotrienes. This leads to damage to the bronchial epithelium, which is responsible for its hyper-reactivity.

Acute asthma may be moderate, severe or life-threatening. Treatment of acute asthma is a medical emergency and should be treated with short-acting β_2 (see later) and systemic prednisolone. Patients with severe or life-threatening asthma should be also given high-flow oxygen and sent immediately to hospital.

In addition to the management of acute asthma exacerbations, therapeutic interventions are also required for the control of chronic asthma. The aims are to control symptoms, prevent exacerbations and maximize pulmonary function.

The British Thoracic Society in conjunction with the Scottish Intercollegiate Guideline Network (BTS and SIGN) have proposed a five-step management plan (see Figure 19.1):

• Step 1 relates to mild asthmatics with intermittent symptoms
• Step 2 for patients with either nocturnal symptoms or more then 3 exacerbations per week
• Step 3 should be initiated if patients continue to experience symptoms despite the first two steps
• Step 4 and Step 5 relate to patients with persistent symptoms

Details of the specific drugs used in this stepwise management of asthma are given later.

Chronic obstructive pulmonary disease (COPD)

COPD is obstructive lung disease caused by irreversible airflow limitation. The term includes those conditions previously referred to as chronic bronchitis and emphysema. It typically presents with a persistent cough, lasting for longer than three months in two years. This is accompanied by an increase in sputum production and eventually shortness of breath. Eventually patients may develop pulmonary hypertension, where there is an increase in pressure within the lung arteries. This increases the workload of the cardiovascular system as may result in heart failure with its associated signs and symptoms.

The main cause of COPD remains tobacco smoking. Other factors implicated include air pollution, occupational exposure to dust, chemicals or fumes and genetic factors. Patients with inherited alpha 1-antitrypsin deficiency are at increased risk of developing COPD.

Although bronchitis and emphysema often co-exist they are the result of different underlying processes. In bronchitis the airways are obstructed as a result of chronic mucosal inflammation, mucous gland hypertrophy and mucus hypersecretion. This is exacerbated by bronchospasm. In emphysema there is progressive destruction of alveolar septa and capillaries leading to enlarged airways and airspaces, decreased lung elastic recoil and increased airway collapsibility. During expiration this leads to collapse of airways and thus airway obstruction. The lungs are hyperinflated increasing respiratory effort.

Exacerbations of COPD are common and can be triggered by lung irritants, such as pollution, or infections, including both viral and bacterial infections. The most frequent bacterial organisms responsible include *Haemophilus influenza* and *Streptococcus pneumonia*.

The management principles for COPD include smoking cessation and avoidance of both the underlying causes as well as triggers to exacerbations, the use of inhaled therapies, similar to those used in asthma and pulmonary rehabilitation. In some patients the use of non-invasive ventilation may be appropriate. Measures to prevent exacerbations should also be instigated.

Rhinitis

Rhinitis is acute or chronic inflammation of the nasal mucosa, which results commonly from viral infections or can be driven by an allergic,

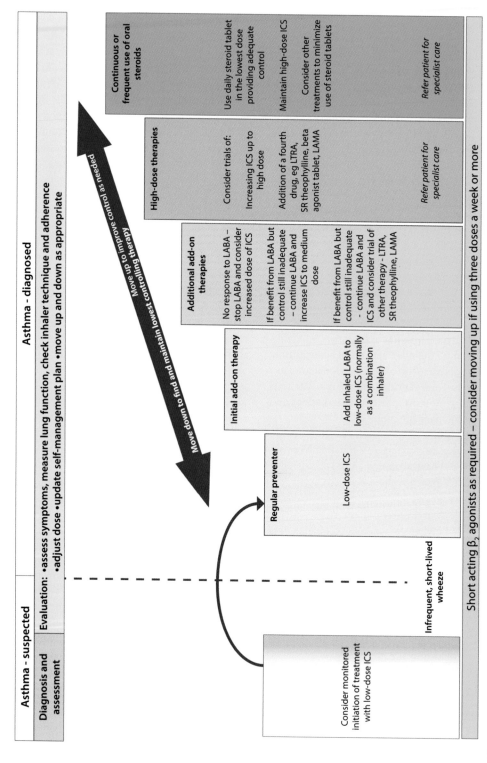

Figure 19.1 The British Thoracic Society/Scottish Intercollegiate Guideline Network five-step asthma management plan.

IgE-mediated reaction that presents as hay fever. Hay fever may be seasonal in response to pollen or perennial in response to ubiquitous allergens. The nasal passages become narrowed due to an increase in nasal mucosal blood flow and permeability causing nasal stuffiness, associated eye irritation and occasionally itchiness of the soft palate. Treatment targets include nasal blood flow with vasoconstrictors, nasal inflammation with glucocorticoids and mediator receptor blockade (both H1 receptor antagonists and leukotriene antagonists) as described later.

Cough

Cough is a symptom rather than a disease entity. It is a common symptom of respiratory infections or may be due to an underlying condition such as asthma or COPD (see earlier), gastro-oesophageal disease, a drug side-effect of ACE inhibitors or it may be due to smoking or allergy.

Over-the-counter cough medications are extremely popular. Antitussives and mucolytics are also sometimes prescribed as discussed later.

Drugs used in respiratory disease

β_2 agonists

β_2-adrenoceptor agonists are bronchodilators. They act directly on β_2-adrenoceptors in bronchial smooth muscle resulting in bronchodilatation. Additionally, they inhibit the release of mediators from mast cells and TNF-α from monocytes, as well as acting on cilia to increase mucus clearance. Their pharmacological effects are brought about by the stimulation of adenylyl cyclase increasing cyclic monophosphate, which in turn phosphorylates a number of enzymes.

Two categories of β_2-adrenoceptor agonists are used in the treatment of obstructive airway disease, short-acting agents and long-acting agents. They are administered by inhalation of an aerosol or a nebulized solution.

Short-acting agents:

Salbutamol is given by inhalation. Approximately 15% enters the respiratory system, where it remains in its free form. The rest is swallowed undergoing presystemic metabolism in the intestine and undergoes hepatic conjugation to inactive metabolites. It reaches its maximum activity within 30 minutes of being administered with duration of action of approximately 4 hours. It is typically used as a 'relieving' inhaler during acute shortness of breath.

Long-acting agents:

Long-acting agents, such as salmeterol and formoterol, are used as 'preventer' drugs to limit acute exacerbations. They not only bind to β_2-adrenoceptors but also to a distinct exo-site where they behave like an irreversible agonist. Salmeterol has a duration of action of 12 hours and is, therefore, taken twice daily.

As β_2-adrenoceptors are found throughout the body their administration can lead to a number of unwanted effects. Most notably their effect on the heart causes an increase in heart rate and force of contraction as well as affecting impulse conduction. This can lead to cardiac dysrhythmias and palpitations. Additionally, they can cause muscle tremors and a dry mouth.

Muscarinic receptor antagonists

Antimuscarinic drugs, such as ipratropium and tiotropium, act on M_2 and M_3 receptors present in bronchi. Both receptors are part of the pathway that ultimately leads to a fall in cAMP and increase in intracellular calcium resulting in bronchoconstriction.

Muscarinc receptor antagonists are administered by aerosol. Ipratropium is a highly polar quaternary nitrogen compound and as such is poorly absorbed systemically when given by inhalation. The maximum effect occurs after 30 minutes and lasts for approximately 4 hours. Tiotropium is a long-acting muscarinc receptor antagonists.

Ipratropium is used in both the prevention and treatment of obstructive lung disease exacerbations. Conversely tiotropium is used in maintenance therapy of patients with COPD.

As muscarinc receptor antagonists are poorly absorbed they have few unwanted systemic effects. However, they can cause urinary retention in patients with prostatic hypertrophy and, when nebulized, acute glaucoma and paradoxical bronchoconstriction (this is due to a preservative in the nebulized solution). Patients often complain about their bitter taste and a dry mouth.

Xanthine drugs

Xanthine drugs include theophylline and theophylline ethylenediamine, also known as aminophylline. The mechanism through which they achieve bronchodilation is not understood. It has been suggested that smooth muscle relaxation may be due to phosphodiesterase isoenzyme inhibition, which results in an increase in cAMP and possibly cGMP. Other possible targets include adenosine A_1 and A_2 receptors where xanthine drugs competitively antagonize adenosine. It is believed they have also have an anti-inflammatory effect and a role in respiratory stimulation in addition to bronchodilation.

Theophylline has a narrow therapeutic range with serious adverse effects reported with minimal increased plasma concentrations. These include cardiac dysrhythmias and seizures, which can be fatal. Close monitoring of plasma concentration is, therefore, required.

Theophylline is given orally whereas aminophylline requires intravenous administration. The half-life is approximately 8 hours. It is metabolized in the liver by P450 enzymes. As a result, its metabolism is significantly affected by drugs that inhibit or induce P450 enzymes. Care is needed when prescribing.

Leukotriene modulators

Cysteinyl leukotriene receptors are expressed in respiratory mucosa and infiltrating inflammatory cells. Montelukast and zafirlukast are cysteinyl leukotriene receptor antagonists. They have a role in the management of exercise-induced asthma and decrease early and late responses to inhaled allergens. Although they do result in a degree of bronchodilation in mild asthma they are used as an adjunct to salbutamol. It is unclear if they have a significant effect on the inflammatory process involved in chronic asthma.

They are often combined with an inhaled corticosteroid. Side effects are rare, however headache and gastrointestinal disturbances have been reported.

Glucocorticoids

Glucocorticoids in asthma and COPD:

Glucocorticoids are used in the management of both asthma, to treat acute exacerbations and prevent progression, and COPD. In asthma glucocorticoids are used as anti-inflammatory agents. Glucocorticoids up-regulate β_2 adrenoceptors, decrease microvascular permeability and reduce cytokine production, particularly those produced by Th2 cells (IL-5 and granulocyte-macrophage colony-stimulating factor), which activate eosinophils and promote both the production of IgE and its effects. By reducing the quantities of IL-3 produced corticosteroids reduce the number of mast cells present in respiratory mucosa. This suppresses the early-phase response to allergens and exercise. In addition COX-2 induction is inhibited through their action on vasodilators PGE_2 and PGI_1

Common inhaled drugs include beclomethasone, budenoside, flucitcasone and mometasone. They must be used for weeks before their full effect is seen. Prednisolone is an oral glucocorticoid.

Glucocorticoids are given in acute exacerbations of COPD although their efficacy is not clear.

Glucocorticoids in rhinitis:

Glucocorticoids applied topically to the nasal mucosa exert an anti-inflammatory effect, reducing nasal congestion and are used in the management of hay fever. Beclomethasone nose drops are effective but encourage excessive dosing and hence may cause adrenal suppression. The main glucocorticoids applied are beclomethasone and fluticasone sprays.

H1 receptor antagonists

H1 receptor antagonists, including cetirizine and fexofenadine, prevent histamine activation of H1 receptors, which is released during an allergic reaction. This reduces inflammation within the nasal mucosa easing ventilation. Since they do not cross the blood-brain barrier, they do not cause drowsiness as does promethazine which is sometimes used for sedation.

α1 adreonceptor agonists

α1 adrenoceptor agonists, such as phenylephrine, produce a degree of vasoconstriction within the nasal mucosa. However their action is not limited to the target site and cause systemic vasoconstriction with resultant changes in blood pressure. Also, they tend to cause rebound nasal stuffiness when discontinued.

Antitussives

Antitussive drugs inhibit the cough reflex. They are used when the cough reflex, normally a protective mechanism, is inappropriately stimulated, for example, as a result of inflammation or neoplasia. Their two broad mechanisms of action are either reducing activation of sensory receptors or acting on the 'cough centre' in the brainstem.

Local anaesthetics, such as topical benzocaine, can be sprayed in order to reduce the activation of 'cough receptors' on the upper airway.

More commonly used antitussive drugs include a number of opioid analgesics which act on the 'cough centre' in the brainstem. Their mechanism of action is little understood. The doses used to suppress cough are lower than those used for analgesia.

Codeine (methylmorphine) is a weak opioid, which reduces bronchial secretions and ciliary activity. Its most problematic side effect is constipation. Morphine is reserved for palliative care. Both can result is respiratory depression. Other examples include pholcodine.

Mucolytics

Normal mucous consists mainly of water with glycoproteins that are cross-linked by disulfide bonds.

A number of conditions result in increased mucus production. Inflammatory exudate additionally binds with glycoproteins to form larger polymers that create a more viscous mucus. In conditions, such as cystic fibrosis, there is a reduction in the ability of the lungs to clear mucus. In both of the above circumstances agents that modify mucus so that it is less viscous can play an important role in their management.

Carbocysteine and mecysteine have free sulfydryl groups that open the disulfide bonds in mucus to reduce its viscosity. They are given orally or by inhalation. The possible unwanted effects include gastrointestinal disturbance and allergic reactions.

Implications for dentistry

For many patients attending for dental treatment can cause significant anxiety. For some patients with respiratory disease, both asthmatics and those with COPD, this can cause an acute exacerbation of their disease. It is, therefore, important to assess both the patient's underlying disease and their feelings towards dentistry. It is advisable to pre-empt any emergency by asking the patient to ensure they bring their own relieving medications with them to appointments and having emergency drugs held within the surgery to be at hand. If the patient should develop acute shortness of breath a β_2-adrenoceptor agonist, salbutamol, should be administered as well as supplemental oxygen. Medical assistance may be required and should be called for early in severe or life-threatening acute exacerbations.

Both patients with asthma and COPD may require systemic corticosteroids to control their disease. It is essential to ask patients with respiratory disease whether or not they are currently taking systemic corticosteroids or indeed if they have recently. This will provide information on the severity or their disease and likelihood or an acute exacerbation. In addition the patient may require corticosteroid cover for treatment in order to prevent an Addisonian crisis.

Inhaled β_2-adrenoceptor agonists and antimuscarinic drugs can cause a dry mouth. This may require symptomatic relief in the form of salivary substitutes as well as causing a number of dental complications, including an increased caries rate and candidosis. They may, therefore, benefit from fluoride supplements and require treatment with antifungal agents. Candidosis may also arise as a result of inhaled corticosteroid use and so patients should ensure they have a good inhaler technique and rinse after inhaler use to minimize the amount of drug present in the mouth.

For a minority of asthmatic patients aspirin and the non-steroidal anti-inflammatory drugs trigger acute exacerbations. Patients should not be prescribed these drugs if there is a history of asthma or any reaction and alternative analgesics should be provided.

CHAPTER 20
Coagulation

Martina Shepard

Key Topics

- Fundamentals of coagulation and haemostasis
- Coagulation disorders
- Platelet function and disorders
- Laboratory investigations
- Considerations in dentistry
- Antiplatelet medications
- Anti-coagulant medications

Learning Objectives

- To understand the process of haemostasis
- To understand the mechanisms of the coagulation cascade
- To understand platelet function
- To identify the most common disorders of haemostasis
- To know how to order and interpret laboratory tests relevant to haemostasis
- To be aware of important considerations in dentistry relating to haemostasis

Essential Dental Therapeutics, First Edition. Edited by David Wray.
© 2018 John Wiley & Sons Ltd. Published 2018 by John Wiley & Sons Ltd.
Companion Website: www.wiley.com/go/wray/dental-therapeutics

Introduction

Coagulation disorders and anti-coagulant therapy are increasingly prevalent among patients with complex medical conditions. There are profound implications for the dental management of such patients. This chapter will consider normal haemostasis followed by consideration of abnormalities affecting platelet function and coagulation disorders in turn. There will then be a consideration of appropriate local measures for control of bleeding and a review of individual anti-coagulant drugs.

Normal haemostasis

The physiology of normal haemostasis will be discussed in the next sub-section followed by a review of the laboratory tests used to assess haemostatic function.

Physiology

Haemostasis refers to the mechanisms by which the body prevents excessive loss of blood from within vessels. There are three major components of haemostasis:

- Local measures such as vasoconstriction
- Primary haemostasis, or formation of a platelet plug
- Secondary haemostasis, known as the coagulation cascade.

Primary haemostasis depends on the presence of sufficient functional platelets to form a platelet plug. Platelets are non-nucleated fragments of megakaryocytes, and are formed in the bone marrow. Their lifespan is 7–10 days and they contain granules filled with hormones, enzymes and other chemicals that are essential for primary haemostasis. The external membrane of the platelet contains glycoproteins, which interact with the vessel wall and other components of the coagulation cascade to assist with haemostasis.

When a vessel wall is damaged, components such as collagen are exposed and platelet glycoproteins contact these surfaces, leading to platelet activation. Following platelet adhesion to an area of damaged vessel either directly or via circulating molecules such as von Willebrand's factor, the platelets are activated, resulting in a change in shape to a more rounded structure, enabling greater surface interactions between platelets. Activation also results in release of platelet granule contents.

Following degranulation, mediators that promote platelet aggregation and adhesion are released leading to the formation of a stable platelet plug to occlude the defect in the vessel. Key mediators include ADP and thromboxane A2, both of which contribute to further platelet adhesion and aggregation. Glycoprotein GPIIb/IIIa will become exposed on the aggregated platelets, and this molecule interacts with the coagulation cascade via the binding of fibrinogen.

The coagulation cascade refers to a sequence of enzyme activation of proteins, with the endpoint being the generation of thrombin. Thrombin converts plasma fibrinogen into fibrin, which forms the basis of the haemostatic plug via interactions with platelets. The coagulation cascade features a number of amplification reactions leading to the generation of sufficient thrombin in order to cause fibrin polymerization and stabilization of the thrombus.

There are two major pathways in the coagulation cascade, known as the extrinsic and intrinsic pathways (Figure 20.1). These converge on the 'common' pathway, which involves the activation of factor X, leading to generation of thrombin, and then the development of fibrinogen. Fibrinogen is hydrolysed by thrombin, releasing peptides that form fibrin monomers, which are then available for polymerization and the formation of a fibrin meshwork, the basis of a blood clot. The initial trigger for coagulation is the interaction of tissue factor (exposed by vascular injury) with clotting factor VII. This starts the extrinsic pathway of coagulation, and leads to activation of factors IX and X, and production of a small amount of thrombin. This pathway is rapidly inactivated by intrinsic anticoagulant functions, so the intrinsic pathway, partially triggered by the small amount of thrombin already produced, takes over and amplifies the coagulation response. This pathway involves a number of coagulation factors and leads to the activation of factors VIII and V. This results in the generation of a larger amount of thrombin, which can then hydrolyse fibrinogen and release fibrin monomers. Polymerization of fibrin,

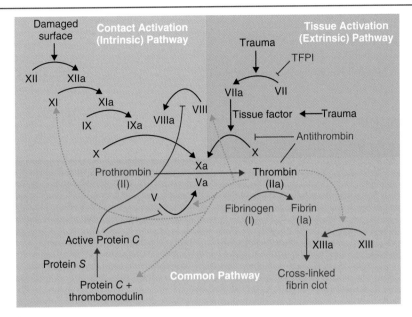

Figure 20.1 The coagulation cascade. *Source*: Medrevise, http://medrevise.co.uk/index.php?title=Coagulation.

assisted by activated factor XIII, leads to the formation of a stable thrombus.

The coagulation process is limited by a number of intrinsic anticoagulants, including tissue factor pathway inhibitor, anti-thrombin, protein C and protein S. The process of fibrinolysis occurs to limit the size of the thrombus developed at a site of vascular injury, and is mediated by plasmin. Plasminogen is converted to plasmin by activators from the vessel wall or tissues. Plasmin will then break down fibrin and thus limit the size of a thrombus, and assists in healing following the vascular injury.

Laboratory investigations

Initial investigations when a bleeding disorder is suspected include a full blood count with differential and a blood film. This may identify a reduction in the platelet count, and the blood film may demonstrate the reason for this, such as haematological malignancy leading to bone marrow failure. Specialized tests are available to assess platelet function.

Investigation of the coagulation system includes tests to assess both the extrinsic and intrinsic pathways.

The prothrombin time (PT) measures the function of factors VII, X, V, prothrombin and fibrinogen (extrinsic pathway). For ease of interpretation and to account for inter-laboratory differences, PT is usually expressed as the international normalized ratio (INR). The INR is a ratio of the patient's PT to a mean normal PT, with a correction in order to calibrate the result against a World Health Organization standard.

Activated partial thromboplastin time (APTT) is used to evaluate the intrinsic coagulation pathway, including factors VIII, IX, XI and XII as well as factors X, V, prothrombin and fibrinogen.

Assays are also available to examine for specific clotting factor deficiencies.

Haemostasis and platelets

As discussed above, platelets are a crucial part of the clotting process and platelet disorders are considered here followed by a discussion of individual antiplatelet drugs.

Platelet disorders

Platelets are produced in the bone marrow by fragmentation of megakaryocyte cytoplasm. The normal platelet count is $150–400 \times 10^9$/L and the average platelet lifespan is approximately 7–10 days.

Platelet disorders encompass abnormalities in the number of platelets as well as their function. Excessive numbers of platelets (thrombocythaemia/thrombocytosis) may be due to a myeloproliferative disorder, or can be reactive following major haemorrhage, as well as in malignancy, chronic infection or connective tissue disorders. Patients who have had their spleen removed may also have elevated platelet counts.

Insufficient platelets (thrombocytopenia) may be due to a failure of production secondary to bone marrow disorders, increased consumption of platelets due to autoimmune disease or other disorders, or sequestration of platelets in the spleen in severe liver disease.

Disorders of platelet function may occur due to hereditary abnormalities of platelet function, in myelodysplastic and myeloproliferative disorders, in patients with renal failure or most commonly, secondary to medications such as aspirin, dipyridamole or clopidogrel.

Considerations in dentistry

Platelet deficiency or impaired platelet function can lead to increased bleeding following oral surgical procedures, due to a failure of primary haemostasis. Typically, formation of the initial blood clot is delayed. Once the clot has formed, haemostasis should be maintained unless there is an additional coagulation defect.

It is now accepted that the risks of cessation of antiplatelet therapy outweigh the small risk of haemorrhage or prolonged bleeding following dental procedures, including simple extractions, and it is no longer recommended that patients stop antiplatelet agents prior to dental treatment. Given the irreversible inhibition caused by drugs such as aspirin, these drugs would need to be ceased 10 days prior to the procedure, so that any circulating platelets affected by the drug are removed from the circulation and replaced by normally functioning platelets. This may lead to an increased risk of thromboembolic disease and the morbidity of these conditions significantly outweighs the small risk of prolonged bleeding following routine dental and oral surgical procedures.

Patients with impaired platelet function secondary to medications should remain on these medications prior to oral surgical procedures, and local measures should be taken to achieve haemostasis. This includes an atraumatic extraction technique, haemostatic suturing, the use of adjuvant agents such as haemostatic dressings (e.g. oxidized cellulose) and medications such as topical tranexamic acid, and the application of pressure. Consideration should be given to carrying out treatment divided over a greater number of appointments (such as extraction of up to only three teeth per session). Patients may need to be monitored for a longer period post-procedure to ensure that haemostasis has been achieved.

Patients with a decreased platelet count due to medical conditions may be at significant risk of major bleeding following oral surgical procedures. Generally, a platelet count below 50×10^9/L is a contraindication to invasive dental treatment, and a platelet transfusion or other measures may be required. Local protocols are available to guide the management of patients requiring oral surgery with platelet counts between $50–150 \times 10^9$/L.

It is recommended that a pre-operative platelet count is reviewed prior to oral surgery in patients with a known haematological malignancy or bone marrow failure due to disease or chemotherapy, in patients with severe liver cirrhosis and/or splenomegaly, and patients with autoimmune platelet disorders.

Antiplatelet drugs

Indications:

Antiplatelet drugs are utilized in situations where there is a high risk of thrombosis formation, due to factors such as damaged blood vessel walls secondary to cardiovascular disease. Their main indication is as secondary prevention in the management of cardiovascular disease, when they are prescribed in order to prevent thrombotic occlusion of coronary arteries and resultant myocardial ischaemia or infarction. Antiplatelet drugs may also be used to reduce the risk of thromboembolic stroke.

Drugs:

Aspirin is an irreversible cyclo-oxygenase inhibitor, leading to inhibition of production of thromboxane A2 and reduced platelet aggregation. Once bound to the platelet the drug is active for the duration of the platelet's life. Aspirin is used at low doses (usually 75 mg daily) for secondary prevention of cardiovascular disease and at high doses (usually 300 mg) in the setting of acute coronary syndromes or ischaemic events.

Clopidogrel is an ADP receptor antagonist, leading to impaired platelet aggregation. It is an irreversible inhibitor of platelet function and remains active for the duration of the life of the platelet. The primary use of this drug is for prevention of thrombosis following coronary stenting and angioplasty, and it may also be used for secondary prevention in cardiovascular disease or following stroke.

Dipyridamole is an adenosine reuptake inhibitor and phosphodiesterase inhibitor. It has a reversible effect on platelet function. It may be prescribed for prophylaxis of thromboembolism associated with prosthetic heart valves, or as secondary prevention of stroke.

Patients with a history of acute coronary syndrome or after coronary stent placement may be prescribed dual antiplatelet therapy, usually a combination of aspirin and clopidogrel.

Coagulation cascade and haemostasis

Secondary haemostasis relies on an intact coagulation cascade. Coagulation disorders can affect any stage of the coagulation cascade, and may be inherited or acquired.

Coagulation disorders

Inherited and acquired coagulation disorders will be discussed in the following sub-sections.

Inherited coagulation disorders:

Inherited coagulation disorders are most commonly due to deficiencies of specific clotting factors. Haemophilia A (factor VIII deficiency), haemophilia B (factor IX deficiency) and von Willebrand disease are the most common inherited coagulation disorders.

In haemophilia A or B, the disease severity is dictated by the percentage of normal coagulation factor activity that is present for the individual patient. Patients with less than 1% normal factor activity will have spontaneous bleeding into joints, muscles and organs. Patients with greater than 5% normal factor activity will have clinically mild disease, with prolonged bleeding after trauma or surgery. These conditions are managed with administration of factor VIII or IX concentrates.

Von Willebrand's disease is the most common inherited coagulopathy, and there are several subtypes. Von Willebrand's factor (VWF) is a molecule involved in platelet adhesion to endothelium, as well as being the carrier molecule for factor VIII, so patients will experience extended bleeding due to failure of the initial haemostatic mechanism as well as the coagulation cascade. The condition is managed by administration of desmopressin or VWF.

Acquired coagulation disorders:

Acquired disorders of coagulation are usually due to a deficiency or functional abnormality of multiple clotting factors. This may be due to vitamin K deficiency, affecting the function of factors II, VII, IX, X and proteins C and S. Deficiency of vitamin K-dependent clotting factors may occur secondary to malabsorption of vitamin K, biliary obstruction, warfarin therapy, and liver disease.

Other causes of acquired coagulopathies include autoantibodies, which may be present in up to 10% of patients with systemic lupus erythematosus. Therapy with heparin or thrombolytic drugs will also alter the function of the coagulation cascade.

Considerations in dentistry

Patients with a significant coagulation disorder are likely to experience prolonged bleeding following oral surgical procedures. Typically, this presents as continued oozing of blood for days to weeks after the procedure, rather than difficulty controlling bleeding immediately following the procedure, as often occurs with platelet disorders.

Pre-operative assessment of coagulation parameters (APTT, INR) is recommended where a bleeding disorder is known or suspected. It is particularly important to consider this in patients with liver disease, as severe liver disease can affect multiple aspects of haemostasis and coagulation, causing platelet deficiency due to splenic sequestration, and failure of hepatic synthesis of clotting factors.

If a known coagulopathy is present, advice should be sought from the patient's treating haematologist prior to oral surgery. Patients with known clotting factor deficiencies will usually have a plan for administration of replacement factor prior to procedures and liaison with their treating physician or clinical nurse specialist will facilitate this.

In general, minor oral surgical procedures may be carried out safely for patients with an INR of up to 4.0. Local haemostatic measures should be used and the patient informed to contact the clinic or attend A&E if prolonged or extensive bleeding occurs.

In patients who have bleeding of unexpectedly long duration following oral surgical procedures, irrigation and re-suturing of the socket, with local haemostatic measures, should be performed for acute control of bleeding. The patient should be referred for investigation of a possible underlying coagulopathy.

Local haemostatic measures

In any patient with an increased risk of bleeding following dental procedures, the same basic management principles apply. Good surgical technique should be used, with a minimally traumatic approach aimed at reducing the amount of tissue disruption and damage. The extent of the procedure may need to be limited, such as performing only one quadrant of deep scaling per visit, or up to three extractions per visit. Following the procedure, local measures to achieve haemostasis should be employed. This includes application of pressure, sometimes for up to 30 minutes, to ensure haemostasis is achieved prior to the patient leaving the surgery. Careful haemostatic suturing is essential. The edges of tissue flaps should be approximated or applied with pressure against a bony surface. Adjuncts such as resorbable collagen sponge or oxidized cellulose can be useful to assist with clot stabilization and achieving primary haemostasis. Some agencies recommend the use of tranexamic acid 5% mouthwash 10 ml four times daily for 5 days following extraction in a patient with an increased bleeding risk. However, there is little evidence to support the use of this medication, and it is not available on the dental formulary so the prescription must be obtained by the patient's GP. The patient should be given very clear post-operative instructions regarding the use of pressure to assist in maintenance of haemostasis, the avoidance of vigorous rinsing to reduce the risk of clot displacement, and when and how to seek further assistance in the case of ongoing bleeding.

Anti-coagulant medications

Indications

Anticoagulation is prescribed for patients at increased risk of thrombotic complications. This may be due to inherited abnormalities such as Factor V Leiden (impaired protein C function), deficiencies of proteins C and S (innate anticoagulants), or abnormal levels of other coagulation factors. Patients with mechanical prosthetic heart valves or atrial fibrillation require lifelong anticoagulation. Risk factors for venous thromboembolism include autoantibodies (such as in lupus erythematosus), oestrogen therapy and pregnancy, immobility especially following major surgery, myeloproliferative disease, malignancy, dehydration, nephrotic syndrome, older age and a history of stroke. Patients with any or a combination of these risk factors may be prescribed anticoagulation for the short or long term. Anticoagulation is used as therapy for 3–6 months following a thrombotic event, such as pulmonary embolism or deep vein thrombosis

(DVT). Prophylactic anticoagulation is usually prescribed for patients undergoing surgical procedures or requiring hospital admission.

Drugs

Coumarins:

The mainstay of oral anticoagulation has been the coumarins, of which the most commonly used drug is warfarin. These drugs are vitamin K antagonists, thereby prolonging coagulation times by inhibiting the function of vitamin K-dependent clotting factors (factors II, VII, XI and X). The anticoagulant effect of warfarin is measured by the INR, and depending on the indication for therapy, a target INR range will be set by the physician. Treatment of DVT or pulmonary embolism, and management of risk factors for thromboembolic disease usually requires a target INR of 2.0–3.0. Mechanical prosthetic heart valves require a target INR of 3.0–4.0.

The metabolism of warfarin is variable between patients and in order to maintain a stable INR in the desired therapeutic range, frequent monitoring of the INR and dose adjustment is required. The dose-response is unpredictable and therapy must be customized to the individual patient, and this often requires frequent dosage adjustments.

Warfarin takes up to 48 hours to be fully active, due to the delay in inhibition of prothrombin, and its mechanism of action relating to liver synthesis of clotting factors.

Warfarin is metabolized in the liver and highly albumin bound, therefore any drugs that affect albumin binding or hepatic/biliary excretion of the drug or its metabolites will have a significant effect on the INR. A large number of drugs interact with warfarin, either potentiating (raising INR) or decreasing (lowering INR) its function. It is important to be aware of the most significant interactions and also to check any prescribed drugs for interactions with warfarin, as the consequences of drug interactions can be extremely serious (haemorrhage or recurrent thrombosis). Drugs commonly prescribed by dentists interact with warfarin, such as azole antifungals and metronidazole, and even topical application of miconazole gel or cream can potentially affect warfarin metabolism and INR.

Dental considerations:

The indications for warfarin therapy are sufficiently serious as to make cessation of warfarin therapy potentially dangerous. As such, it is essential that the drug is not ceased for dental procedures. If warfarin cessation is required for a high bleeding-risk procedure, this must be done in conjunction with the treating physician and 'bridging therapy' with an alternative anticoagulant such as heparin is arranged, usually on an inpatient basis.

The British Committee for Standards in Haematology advise that simple extractions may be carried out safely with an INR up to 4.0. It is recommended that an INR reading is obtained within 72 hours of a planned extraction, and the procedure postponed if the INR is above 4.0. Patients with an unstable INR should have the level checked within 24 hours of the procedure, and liaison with the patient's GP or treating specialist will facilitate this process. Use of local haemostatic strategies are essential for control of bleeding. The patient should be monitored and clear post-operative advice given for actions to take in case of prolonged or excessive bleeding.

Novel anticoagulants

New oral anticoagulants (dabigatran, rivaroxaban, apixaban) target specific clotting factors, leading to a more predictable dose response than warfarin. They do not require monitoring and dose adjustments, have no food or medication interactions, and have a number of other potential advantages over warfarin therapy. However, the majority of these drugs lack a reversal agent, which can lead to potentially fatal major haemorrhage, and there is a relative lack of clinical experience in their use.

Dabigatran:

Dabigatran is a direct thrombin inhibitor. Clot formation is impaired as the lack of active thrombin inhibits the conversion of fibrinogen to fibrin. Thrombin is also involved in the activation of factors V, VIII and XI so the drug further affects coagulation via this mechanism. Dabigatran is used for prophylaxis of thromboembolic events in patients with atrial fibrillation (AF). It is given at a fixed dose and does not require regular monitoring. On laboratory investigations APTT is prolonged however INR does not change significantly.

Rivaroxaban and Apixaban:

Rivaroxaban and apixaban are factor Xa inhibitors and may be used for stroke prevention in AF, and for treatment and prevention of pulmonary embolism and DVT. Again, they are given at fixed doses and do not require monitoring.

Dental considerations:

These drugs have a shorter half-life than warfarin and are renally excreted, so in patients with normal renal function the timing of oral surgical procedures can be managed to reduce the risk of bleeding. It is suggested that procedures are carried out 18–24 hours after the last dose of these drugs – this may mean that one dose of the medication is missed or delayed, however current guidance suggests that this is acceptable.

For patients continuing to take novel anticoagulants, it is considered safe to carry out procedures with no clinically significant bleeding risk, including up to three simple extractions, periodontal surgery, incision and drainage of an abscess, and implant placement. In these situations, additional local haemostatic measures and post-operative tranexamic acid 5% mouthwash (10 ml four times daily for 5 days) may be used. Again, careful follow-up is necessary and post-operative instructions should be given.

If a procedure with a high risk of bleeding is to be undertaken, careful consideration needs to be given to the risk of cessation of anticoagulant therapy. This decision should be made in conjunction with the patient's treating physician. In cases where the bleeding risk is considered significant, calculations based on creatinine clearance may be made in order to guide how far in advance of surgery the drug needs to be stopped. This should only be done in conjunction with the patient's physician given the risks of ceasing anticoagulation.

Heparins

Heparin activates antithrombin, which then irreversibly binds to a number of coagulation factors, rendering them inactive. It also impairs platelet function. Heparins are not absorbed from the gastrointestinal tract so they are given via intravenous or subcutaneous routes. Standard heparin is usually administered by continuous infusion in an inpatient setting.

Low molecular weight heparin (LMWH) inhibits factor Xa more significantly than standard heparin and has fewer effects on platelets. These drugs have a longer half-life and are administered subcutaneously. They have a more predictable effect and require less monitoring than standard heparin.

LMWH is used for prevention of DVT, particularly in peri-operative or hospital settings. It may also be used for treatment of PE and acute coronary syndromes. Once daily LWMH is prescribed for DVT prophylaxis and twice daily for treatment of existing thrombosis. Patients may self-administer LMWH therapy subcutaneously so it is important to ask specifically about this as part of the medical history prior to dental treatment.

Heparin therapy is monitored using APTT. APTT is usually maintained at 1.5–2.5 times the upper limit of normal. Anti-Xa levels may be used to monitor LMWH therapy although monitoring is not usually required.

Dental considerations:

Patients receiving heparin infusions will be hospital inpatients and non-urgent dental procedures should usually be postponed. Patients requiring procedures with a significant bleeding risk and who are warfarinized may be admitted to hospital and placed on heparin bridging therapy to facilitate the procedure. These situations should be managed by specialists in oral surgery in conjunction with the patient's treating physician.

Patients receiving LMWH on an outpatient basis may require dental treatment involving a risk of bleeding. There is little clinical evidence regarding bleeding risks associated with dental treatment for patients on these medications, and specialist advice should be sought prior to invasive dental treatment.

CHAPTER 21

Gastrointestinal pharmacology

Esther Hullah

Key Topics

- Overview
- Gastric acid-related conditions
- Anti-emetics
- Diarrhoea and constipation
- Inflammatory bowel disease

Learning Objectives

- To understands the key anatomical components of the gastrointestinal tract and their relevant pharmacology
- To have knowledge of the common side effects of drugs acting on the gastrointestinal tract and their relevance to prescribing in dentistry
- To be aware of importance of immunosuppression in inflammatory bowel disease and its relevance to dentistry

Essential Dental Therapeutics, First Edition. Edited by David Wray.
© 2018 John Wiley & Sons Ltd. Published 2018 by John Wiley & Sons Ltd.
Companion Website: www.wiley.com/go/wray/dental-therapeutics

Introduction

The gastrointestinal tract's (GIT) main function is that of digestion and absorption of food. It is also one of the major endocrine systems of the body. There is a wide range of gastrointestinal disorders that have oral manifestations and impact on a patient's oral health.

The GIT and its relevant pharmacology can be divided into the stomach and gastric acid-related conditions, management of nausea and vomiting, constipation and diarrhoea, irritable bowel syndrome, the management of inflammatory bowel disease and the medical management of gallstones. There are also many drugs that adversely affect gastrointestinal function (see Table 21.1).

Gastric acid-related conditions

Gastric acid has many purposes including providing an optimal environment for proteolytic enzymes to work and improving the sterility of the stomach contents. It is controlled by local and systemic endocrine effects.

Acid secretion from parietal cells is increased by:

- Acetyl choline from the vagus nerve
- Histamine from local nerve endings acting on histamine type II receptors
- Gastrin secreted by the antrum of the stomach.

The exact mechanism of action of these three stimulants on the parietal cell is unclear.

Acid secretion is decreased by:

- Prostaglandin receptors on the luminal surface of the cell.

Table 21.1 Gastrointestinal conditions requiring medical management
Gastric acid-related conditions
Nausea and vomiting
Constipation
Diarrhoea
Irritable bowel syndrome
Inflammatory bowel disease
Gallstones

All of these mechanisms work on the 'proton pump' and gastrin provides a negative feedback: an acid environment in the stomach decreases gastrin output thus shutting down acid secretion.

Peptic ulcers

In peptic ulceration there is an imbalance in the protective elements (mucus secretion, gastric blood flow) and harmful elements (acid, exotoxins, drugs). Complications include pain, anaemia, severe bleeding, perforation and pyloric stenosis (caused by fibrosis following inflammation).

Duodenal ulcers:

Duodenal ulcers are often associated with high acid output and *Helicobacter pylori* infection. They have no malignant potential. They can be cured by acid suppression but have a high recurrence rate. This can be reduced by eradication of *H. pylori*.

Gastric ulcers:

These are often associated with low or normal acid output and the use of non-steroidal anti-inflammatory drugs. They are sometimes related to *H. pylori* infection. They have a risk of malignant transformation.

Medications used in gastric acid-related conditions

Antacids

These reduce gastric acidity and thus diminish the activity of gastric pepsin. They can relieve the pain of peptic ulceration; however they do not promote healing unless large doses are given frequently. Antacids are generally not toxic, but large doses can lead to side effects: sodium bicarbonate in large doses can cause alkalosis and calcium carbonate in excess can induce hypercalcaemia. For this reason, magnesium and aluminium compounds are preferred such as magnesium carbonate and aluminium hydroxide.

Helicobactor pylori eradication

H. pylori is spread by the faeco-oral route. It is associated with over 95% of duodenal ulcers and

70% of gastric ulcers. *H. Pylori* colonizes the antrum of the stomach, where it secretes urease, creating an alkaline microenvironment to protect itself. It interferes with normal control of acid secretion and also secretes exotoxins which directly damage the mucosa. Eradication of *H. pylori* can be achieved using a combination of a proton pump inhibitor (e.g. omeprazole) and two antibiotics (e.g. clarithromycin and amoxicillin).

Acid secretion reducing drugs
Histamine receptor antagonists:

These drugs, such as cimetidine and ranitidine, work as histamine antagonists at H2 receptors. They decrease acid secretion and aid in healing duodenal ulcers. They can be used in the treatment of reflux oesophagitis and they relieve symptoms of dyspepsia.

These drugs have several adverse effects: cimetidine has a weak anti-androgen effect and can cause gynaecomastia in long-term use. They can cause confusion and drowsiness particularly in the elderly. Cimetidine is a liver enzyme inhibitor and may increase the effects and toxicity of other drugs.

Proton pump inhibitors:

These drugs, such as omeprazole or lansoprazole, irreversibly inhibit the H+/K+ ATPase enzyme (proton pump) and so reduce acid secretion. They aid healing of acid-related disorders. They may be used long term in reflux oesophagitis and in high doses they are used in the treatment of Zollinger-Ellison syndrome. Side effects include headache, nausea, vomiting and diarrhoea.

Mucosal protectants

These drugs help to enhance the protective elements of the mucosa so allowing healing to occur.

Sucralfate:

Sucralfate polymerizes at low pH to give a very sticky gel that adheres strongly to the base of ulcer craters. Bismuth chelate acts in a similar way to sucralfate. It has affinity for mucosal glycoproteins, particularly in the necrotic tissue of an ulcer so it becomes coated in a protective layer of polymer-glycoprotein complex. They must be given on an empty stomach or else will complex with food proteins. In addition, Bismuth can blacken teeth and stools.

Nausea and vomiting

Nausea and vomiting are common, non-specific features of disease or drug toxicity and it is important to establish the underlying cause and give specific treatment if possible.

Vomiting is caused by activation of the vomiting centre in the brainstem, mainly through activation of the vagus nerve. The vomiting centre is also influenced by the vestibular apparatus, the cerebral cortex, afferents from the GIT and by the chemoreceptor trigger zone, through muscarinic and histamine (H1) receptors. The chemoreceptor trigger zone is another region of the brainstem and is activated by afferents (often D2 doperminergic) similar to those of the vomiting centre. In addition it is activated by toxins, including drugs.

Anti-emetics

Anti-emetics, discussed in the following subsections, act in several different ways.

Anticholinergic drugs

These drugs, such as hyoscine, act on the vomiting centre in particular but also may affect the gastrointestinal tract directly. They may cause a dry mouth or agitation.

Antihistamines

These drugs, such as promethiazine, act on H1 receptors in the vomiting centre and also have weak anticholinergic and sedating effects.

Phenothiazines

These drugs, such as prochlorperazine, have anticholinergic, sedative, H1 blocking and dopamine receptor antagonist activity in the chemoreceptor trigger zone.

Dopamine receptor antagonists

These drugs, such as metoclopramide, act in the chemoreceptor trigger zone and have a direct effect on the GIT.

Adverse effects include extrapyramidal actions such as oculogyric crisis. Increased prolactin concentrations and gynaecomastia can occur in prolonged use.

Domperidone

This is similar to metoclopramide but is less likely to cause extrapyramidal reactions. It can however cause cardiac arrhythmias when given parenterally in high dose.

5-Hydroxytryptamine (5-HT) antagonists

These drugs, such as ondansetron, are very effective in severe nausea when other drugs have proved ineffective. Their side effects include constipation and headache.

Corticosteroids

Corticosteroids, such as dexamethasone, are useful anti-emetics in anti-cancer treatment or terminal illness.

Constipation

Constipation can be treated effectively with dietary modification including increased fibre and water intake.

Bulking agents

Bulking agents, such as bran or ispaghula, absorb water, swell and increase the bulk of the stool which stimulates peristalsis and hence defaecation. Adverse effects include flatulence and abdominal cramps. They may take a few days to act.

Osmotic laxatives

Osmotic laxatives, such as lactulose, reduce reabsortion of water from the bowel, so increasing bulk and stimulating peristalsis. They may cause abdominal pain and flatulence.

Stimulants

Stimulants, such as senna, castor oil and bisacodyl, stimulate peristalsis and have a rapid effect (within 8 hours). Long-term use is inadvisable due to possible bowel atony.

Faecal softeners

Faecal softeners, like liquid paraffin, lubricate and soften stool.

Diarrhoea

Diarrhoea is common and has many causes. It is essential, especially in children, to replace fluid and electrolyte losses. As most cases of diarrhoea are self-limiting, specific anti-diarrhoeal drugs are often not necessary.

Anti-motility drugs

These drugs, such as loperamide and diphenoxylate, stimulate opioid receptors in the bowel and reduce peristalsis. They may cause constipation.

Adsorbents

These drugs, such as kaolin, absorb water without increasing stool bulk, so the stool if firmer and smaller.

Infective diarrhoea

In infective diarrhoea it is essential is to replace fluid and electrolyte losses. Drugs to reduce intestinal mobility are contraindicated. Severe bacterial diarrhoea can be treated with an appropriate antibiotic, commonly trimethoprim or ciprofloxacin. Erythromycin or ciprofloxacin are given for campylobacter infection, a common cause of diarrhoea.

Irritable bowel syndrome

Irritable bowel syndrome is caused by dysmotility of the bowel. Symptoms may include intermittent diarrhoea and constipation, and abdominal pain. Drug treatment is symptomatic.

Antispasmodics

These drugs, such as mebeverine or propantheline, have anticholinergic activity and decrease bowel motility by reducing peristalsis and treat painful spasms of the large bowel.

Inflammatory bowel disease

This includes Ulcerative colitis, which affects the large bowel and Crohn's disease, which can affect any part of the gastrointestinal tract from mouth to anus. Both diseases can undergo exacerbations and remissions. Treatment is aimed at resolving acute episodes and prolonging remissions. Treatment may also involve correction of nutritional deficiencies and possible surgery for complications or severe uncontrolled disease.

Crohn's disease

Crohn's disease is a chronic inflammatory condition and has a particular tendency to affect the terminal ileum and ascending colon (ilieocolonic). The disease can involve one area of the gut such as the terminal ileum or multiple areas with relatively normal bowel in between (skip lesions). It may also involve the whole of the colon (total colitis) sometimes without small bowel involvement. Macroscopic changes include deep ulcers and fissures in the mucosa producing a cobblestone appearance. Fistulae and abscess may be seen. If the face and oral cavity is involved it is part of the spectrum of Oro-facial Granulomatosis (OFG). OFG may present with lip swelling extra-orally and intra-orally, sulcal ulceration, mucosal tags and cobblestoning. Crohn's isolated to the lips and oral cavity often responds well to a cinnamon and benzoate exclusion diet.

Ulcerative colitis

Ulcerative colitis can affect the rectum alone (proctitis), can extend proximally to involve the sigmoid and descending colon (left-sided colitis), or may involve the whole colon (total colitis). Sometimes there may be inflammation of the distal terminal ileum (backwash ileitis). Macroscopically, the mucosa looks reddened, inflamed and bleeds easily.

In severe disease there is extensive ulceration with the adjacent mucosa appearing as inflammatory polyps.

Drugs used in inflammatory bowel disease

Several types of drugs are used in the management of inflammatory bowel disease.

Corticosteroids:

These may be used in acute episodes and can be given rectally, orally or intravenously depending on the extent and severity of the condition. Rectal steroids can be given in mild to moderate attacks of ulcerative colitis limited to the left side of the colon. In more severe or extensive cases, oral prednisolone should be given. The dose of prednisolone can be reduced as symptoms improve, and ultimately stopped.

Steroid-sparing agents:

Other anti-inflammatories, such as Azathioprine or Ciclosporin, are often used to maintain remission of disease.

Azathioprine is a pro-drug and is metabolized to 6-mercaptopurine which undergoes metabolism to various active metabolites (thioguanine nucleotides). Thioguanine nucleotides are incorporated into DNA and have an anti-proliferative effect, especially on lymphocytes, giving its immunosuppressive activity, and on other haemopoietic cells. The principal deactivating pathways are regulated by the enzymes thiopurine methyltransferase (TPMT) and xanthine oxidase. Impairment of these pathways, due to inherent low enzyme activity or drug interactions (for example with allopurinol which blocks the actions of xanthine oxidase) can lead to accumulation of potentially toxic levels of thioguanine nucleotides and the risk of life-threatening bone marrow suppression. It is essential to measure the TPMT activity prior to commencing Azathioprine. The action of onset is slow and therapeutic effects can take several months. Appropriate haematological and biochemical serology is required throughout treatment. Dose escalation minimizes side effects such as nausea and the target dose range is usually 1–3 mg/kg. Thioguanine nucleotide levels can be monitored during therapy to ascertain if patients are within the ideal therapeutic range, and necessary dose adjustment can be made. Adverse effects include gastrointestinal upset, hypersensitivity, hepatitis, haematological abnormalities, including bone marrow suppression, infections, pancreatitis and an increased risk of malignancy including non-melanoma skin cancer.

Biological agents:

Infliximab is a chimeric monoclonal antibody which inhibits the action of inflammatory cytokine tumour necrosis factor (TNF) alpha. It is used in refractory Crohn's disease. Adalimumab is a human monoclonal antibody which binds to TNF alpha receptor and is also of the use in refractory disease.

Aminosalicylates:

Sulfasalazine is a complex of a sulfonamide, sulfapyridine, and 5-aminosalicylate (5-ASA). It can be taken orally or rectally and is broken down by bacteria to release 5-ASA. Sulfapyridine is absorbed into the circulation and is metabolized by the liver.

In relapses of ulcerative colitis or Crohn's disease, sulfasalazine is given with systemic corticosteroids. It can also be given to maintain remission.

Adverse effects include nausea, vomiting, headache and skin rashes.

Mesalazine is a controlled release preparation of 5-ASA, which is released in the terminal ileum and colon. It lacks the side effects attributed to sulfapyridine in sulfasalazine.

Gallstones

In the developed world, gallstones are usually made of cholesterol. Bile acids maybe used to dissolve cholesterol gallstones. Treatment for 3–6 months is required and recurrence is common. This treatment is generally reserved for patient for whom surgery is contraindicated. These drugs include chenodeoxyxholic acid, and ursodeoxycholic acid which may cause diarrhoea.

CHAPTER 22

Antineoplastic therapeutics

Jenny Taylor and John Steele

Key Topics

- Introduction
- Chemotherapy
- Hormone therapy
- Biological therapy
- Transplants
- Bisphosphonates
- Other treatments

Learning Objectives

- To be familiar with the various therapeutic agents used in the management of cancer
- To be aware of the various oral adverse effects related to anti neoplastic treatments
- To understand the role of the dentist during cancer treatment

Essential Dental Therapeutics, First Edition. Edited by David Wray.
© 2018 John Wiley & Sons Ltd. Published 2018 by John Wiley & Sons Ltd.
Companion Website: www.wiley.com/go/wray/dental-therapeutics

Introduction

A neoplasm is a new and abnormal growth of cells. A malignant neoplasm, more commonly known as cancer, has the potential to invade and spread throughout the body.

Management of cancer has traditionally focused on a trio of potential treatments including chemotherapy, surgery and radiotherapy; however, the area of antineoplastic therapeutics is rapidly progressing. Advanced new treatments are being developed to direct treatments in a more defined way. These include hormone therapies, biological therapies and bisphosphonates.

The number of patients surviving and living with cancer is increasing and many of these patients will be under the care of the oncology team and may be prescribed long-term antineoplastic therapies. The traditional intravenous inpatient 'chemotherapy' is still an important part of cancer management. However, a number of new medications for cancer now allow patients to self-administer treatments at home. These patients may not think of their medications as 'chemotherapy' especially those patients on oral tablet treatment, however it is essential that dentists are fully aware of all the drugs the patient may be taking due to the potential impact on oral health and interactions with dental prescribing.

This chapter will give a brief overview of the currently known therapeutics available for cancer (Table 22.1).

Chemotherapy (cytotoxic therapeutics)

Chemotherapy literally translated means treatment with drugs, but in cancer, chemotherapy describes

Table 22.1 The currently known therapeutics available for cancer

Chemotherapy
Hormone therapy
Biological therapy
Transplants
Bisphosphonates
Other treatments

Table 22.2 Generic side effects of cytotoxic drugs

Adverse reproductive function
Alopecia
Bone marrow suppression
Gastrointestinal (nausea and vomiting)
Hyperuricaemia
Oral mucositis
Tumour lysis syndrome

the use of cytotoxic treatments. There are over 100 different cytotoxic drugs available for cancer treatment. Patients can be treated with both individual and combination regimes.

There are a number of generic side effects that are commonly associated with cytotoxic drugs. These are listed in Table 22.2.

These side effects, in turn, may be managed by a range of specific agents, for example, folinic acid is used to counter the effects of methotrexate which is a folic acid antagonist (see Table 22.3).

Cytotoxic therapeutics can be divided into the drug types shown in Table 22.4.

Table 22.3 Therapeutics used to prevent and treat the side effects of cytotoxic drugs

Amifostine for chemotherapy-induced neutropenic infection and nephrotoxicity
Dexrazoxane to treat anthracycline side effects
Folinic acid for chemotherapy-induced mucositis and myelosuppression
Levofolonic acid for chemotherapy-induced mucositis and myelosuppression
Mesna to prevent urothelial toxicity (given with cyclophosphamide, ifosfamide)
Palifermin for chemotherapy-induced mucositis and myelosuppression

Table 22.4 Cytotoxic therapeutics

Alkylating drugs
Cytotoxic antibiotics
Antimetabolites
Vinca alkaloids/etoposide

Alkylating drugs

These are the most commonly used cytotoxic drugs. They work by causing damage to the DNA within the cell which stops the cell from replicating. The main action is on rapidly proliferating cells leading to a depletion of B and T cell lymphocytes and suppression of both cell-mediated immunity and antibody production.

The main problems encountered with prolonged use of this group of drugs are teratogenicity and an increase in the incidence of acute non-lymphoblastic leukaemia (especially when treatment is combined with radiotherapy). The more common alkylating drugs are shown in Table 22.5. Cisplatin, an alkylating-like drug, is particularly used in testicular and ovarian cancers.

Cytotoxic antibiotics (including anthracyclines)

A wide variety of cancers can be treated with this group of medications. These include non-Hodgkin's B cell lymphoma, advanced ovarian cancer, acute leukaemias, upper gastrointestinal, breast and bladder cancers. These antibiotics are listed in Table 22.6.

There are many drug specific adverse events relating to individual treatments including mucositis, myelosuppression and hyperpigmentation of skin, nails and oral mucosa. Toxicity can be increased with concomitant use of radiotherapy.

Table 22.5 Alkylating drugs

Bendamustine
Busulfan
Carmustine
Chloarambucil
Cyclophosphamide
Estramustine
Ifosamide
Lomustine
Melphalan
Mitobronitol
Thiopeta
Treosulfan

Table 22.6 Cytotoxic and Anthracycline antibiotics

Cytotoxic antibiotics	Anthracycline antibiotics
Bleomycin	Daunorubicin
Dactinomycin	Doxorubicin
Mitomycin	Epirubicin
Mitoxantrone	Idarubicin
Pixantrone	

Antimetabolites

Antimetabolites have two main modes of action. They can work by becoming part of the nuclear material or they can combine with the cell enzymes causing irreversible abnormal cellular division.

For these reasons, they can be used in a range of cancers (leukaemias, lymphomas and various solid tumours) both as mono therapy and combined therapies. Table 22.7 lists some of the major antimetabolites.

Vinca alkaloids/etoposide

This group of treatments can be used to treat a range of cancers including leukaemias, lymphomas and

Table 22.7 Antimetabolites

Azacitidine
Capecitabine
Cladribine
Clofarabine
Cytarabine
Decitabine
Fludarabine
Fluorouracil
Gemcitabine
Mercaptopurine
Methotrexate
Nelarabine
Pemetrexed
Raltitrexed
Tegafur
Tioguanine

Table 22.8 Vinca alkaloids
Etoposide
Vinblastine
Vincristine
Vindesine
Vinflunine

various solid tumours. The most common adverse event with this group of drugs is the development of neurotoxicity (both autonomic and peripheral neuropathy) which occurs with all vinca alkaloids. Vinca alkaloids are listed in Table 22.8.

Hormone therapy

Various cancers use hormones to progress and are known as hormone receptive or hormone sensitive cancers. Hormone treatments can be used as a way of suppressing the growth of cancers or preventing recurrence. Table 22.9 lists some hormone therapies.

Biological therapy

This is a rapidly evolving and complex area of cancer management. There are a wide variety of therapies available with a multitude of individual actions. As such, there is no simple classification process. The decision to use a biological therapy depends not only on the primary cancer type, but also on the staging of the cancer and what previous treatments have been used. Due to the expense of many of the treatments, their use in the NHS in England and Wales is regulated via NICE guidelines. Oncology departments often invite patients to take part in large scale clinical trials. However, these often have significant inclusion and exclusion criteria meaning that for the patients with the most advanced disease and the most complex previous therapy history, treatment with the most advanced new discoveries is not a possibility.

Monoclonal antibodies

Monoclonal antibodies are laboratory produced antibodies that are used as targeted antineoplastic treatments. These are designed to recognize and attach themselves to specific proteins, which are produced by various cell types. These medications usually end in -mab.

General side effects can include fever, rash and shortness of breath.

Anti-angiogenesis treatments

Anti-angiogenesis treatments work by inhibiting the blood supply to the cancer cells. This is achieved in three main ways

- by blocking the blood vessel growth factor,
- inhibiting intracellular messaging, and
- stopping intercellular signalling.

Examples of anti-angiogenesis inhibitors are shown in Table 22.10.

The most 'significant to dentistry' adverse effect of this group of treatments is the risk of osteonecrosis of the jaw. If possible, invasive dental procedures should be avoided in patients on sunitinib or bevacuzimab.

Interferon and interleukin 2

Interferon and interleukin 2 are cytokines used in intercellular communication. These treatments work by interfering with the growth of cancer cells and by stimulating the host immune response. They are often used in myeloma, melanoma and renal cell carcinoma. Fatigue, nausea and flu like symptoms are common side effects.

Gene therapy

There is ongoing research in this area including clinical trials of newly developed gene-therapy treatments. To enable the entry of genes into the cancer cells various vectors are used including the use of viruses and inactivated bacteria. An example is the use of a treatment called *oncovex* which uses the herpes simplex virus to help treat melanoma and pancreatic cancer. It is also a promising area for treatment of head and neck cancers which are generally poorly responsive to chemotherapy.

Vaccines

Vaccines can be used to either prevent cancer or treat cancer.

Table 22.9 Hormone therapies

Oestrogens	Diethylstilbestrol	Breast Prostate
	Ethinylestradiol	Prostate (palliative)
Progestogens	Medroxyprogesterone Megestrol Norithesterone	Endometrial Breast, renal prostate (rarely)
Hormone antagonists	Anastrozole Letrozole Exemestane Trastuzumab Fulvestrant Tamoxifen Toremifene	Breast
Gonadorelin analogues	Buserelin Goserelin Histrelin Leuprorelin acetate Triptorelin	Prostate Breast
Anti-androgens	Abiraterone acetate Bicalutamide Cyproterone acetate Enzalutamide Flutamide	Prostate
Gonadotrophin-releasing hormone antagonists	Degarelix	Prostate
Somatostatin analogues	Lanreotide	Neuroendocrine tumours Thyroid
	Octreotide	Neuroendocrine tumours Post pancreatic resection Antiemetic in palliative care

Table 22.10 Examples of anti-angiogenesis inhibitors

Blocking the blood vessel growth factor (VEGF vascular endothelial growth factor)	Bevacuzimab (Avastin) used in breast, colorectal and ovarian cancers
Inhibition of intracellular messaging (includes tyrosine kinase inhibitors TKIs whose names usually end in -nib))	Sunitinib (sutent) used in kidney cancer and gastrointestinal stromal tumours
Modulation of intercellular signalling	Thalidomide used for myeloma

Prevention:

HPV 16 and 18 (human papilloma virus) is closely linked to cervical cancer and anal cancer and more recently to oropharyngeal cancers. Large scale vaccination programmes have been ongoing vaccinating young girls aged 11 or 12. In some countries young boys are also vaccinated.

Treatment:

The current vaccines work by stimulating the immune system to attack the cancer cells. It is an innovative and new area of therapy. There are a small number of trials ongoing.

The Bacillus Calmette-Guerin (BCG) vaccine, which is used to prevent tuberculosis, is also an effective adjunct treatment following surgery for some non-invasive bladder cancers. It is given directly into the bladder.

Transplants

Bone marrow or stem cell transplants can be used to treat myeloproliferative diseases such as leukaemia, lymphoma and myeloma.

Bone marrow transplant

Bone marrow is found inside bones and is responsible for creating blood cells. Prior to whole-body radiation, the patient's own bone marrow can be harvested for use at a later stage. Alternatively donated bone marrow can be used. This should be carefully and closely HLA matched to the recipient. Graft versus host disease (GVHD) is caused by the immune system responding to the graft and it is more common in bone marrow transplants than stem cell transplants. Advanced GVHD can be catastrophic, but it is thought that a low level of GVHD is a good sign as it represents a responsive immune system which attempts to 'mop up' any remaining cancer cells. GVHD can present with oral lesions which mimic oral lichen planus or a lichenoid reaction. These are thought to be potentially malignant lesions due to the long-term, drug-induced, immunosuppression of the patients. These patients should be closely monitored for any worrying oral changes.

Stem cell transplants

Stem cells are the essential precursor blood cells that develop in the bone marrow to form red blood cells, white blood cells and platelets. Transplants can be collected from the patient themselves (after growth factor therapy) or from a donor. It is important that donated cells are a close HLA match. This is more likely when a sibling or close relative donates. Mismatch can lead to an exaggerated graft versus host disease leading to multiple side effects and possibly rejection.

It is important for dentists to be aware of any previous transplants as the patient will be on a number of immunosuppressant treatments.

This will affect not only dental prescribing, but also long-term dental management of any potential infective dental problems.

Bisphosphonates

There are a variety of indications for the use of bisphosphonates. The most common one is for prevention and treatment of osteoporosis. This is often given as a low dose, oral treatment. In cancer therapy much higher doses are used and often by the intravenous route. The aim is to treat bone cancer and to prevent any weakening of the bones secondary to cancer or cancer treatments. They are used in cancers such as myeloma, lung and breast. Examples include disodium pamidronate (aredia) and zoledronic acid (zometa).

It is essential for dentists to be aware if a patient is on a bisphosphonate due to the risk of bisphosphonate related osteonecrosis of the jaw (BRONJ). Often patients forget they are on a bisphosphonate as it can be a weekly, or in some cases, yearly injection. High dose bisphosphonates are much more likely to cause BRONJ although the risk is still increased in those taking low doses.

Other treatments

Corticosteroids

Corticosteroids can be given to enhance the effects of cancer treatments or reduce the side effects of treatments. They are also often given to stimulate appetite.

Analgesics

A variety of analgesic treatments are available. In particular opioids are used in often large dosages. These opioids can be given in a variety of ways such as orally (tablet, liquid or 'lollypop'), dermal patches, subcutaneous or intramuscular injections or intravenously. Neuropathic painkillers such as gabapentin and pregabalin can also be used for nerve related pain.

The oral adverse effect is dry mouth which should be managed appropriately with prevention and lubrication.

Combination therapy

Combining various treatments is a very common approach to treating cancer.

There are various acronyms used to describe common combinations, for example CHOP (**C**yclophosphamide, doxorubicin (**h**ydroxydaunomycin), Vincristine (**O**ncovin®), **P**rednisolone).

Dental management of the patient undergoing treatment for cancer

It is important to manage these patients actively throughout their cancer journey. At diagnosis thought should be given to an early dental check up to identify and treat any potential dental problems. Areas of chronic sepsis can flare as a result of immunosuppression and so potential dental problems should ideally be managed before cancer therapy begins. Also, many of the patients will be very unwell during the acute stages of treatment and may be unable to attend a dental practice. If they do manage to attend, they may have evidence of oral mucositis, ulceration, candidosis or a profoundly dry mouth either as a result of chemotherapy or radiotherapy. Following the initial stages of cancer treatment, the dentist should be kept informed of current medications including corticosteroids, immunosuppression, angiogenesis inhibitors or bisphosphonates as these have a direct impact on dental care.

CHAPTER 23

Vitamins and minerals

Sabine Jurge

Key Topics

- Overview of role of micronutrients
- Water and fat soluble vitamins
- Minerals and trace elements

Learning Objectives

- To be able to list different vitamins and minerals
- To be able to explain their role in human health including the oral health

Essential Dental Therapeutics, First Edition. Edited by David Wray.
© 2018 John Wiley & Sons Ltd. Published 2018 by John Wiley & Sons Ltd.
Companion Website: www.wiley.com/go/wray/dental-therapeutics

Introduction

Micronutrients, such as vitamins and minerals, have an important role in maintaining general and oral health. There are several reasons why people take vitamins and minerals. These can be prescribed by doctors to treat a deficiency: vitamin B_{12} intramuscular injections are used to manage pernicious anaemia; iron preparations are used to manage iron deficiency. They may also be used to prevent a disease, for example calcium and vitamin D supplements can be used in certain patient groups to prevent osteoporosis and folate supplements are recommended for pregnant women to prevent neural tube pathologies in the foetus.

Sometimes vitamin preparations are used to treat a disease that is not caused by underlying vitamin deficiency, for example the use of vitamin A in treatment of severe acne or psoriasis. In addition, people often take vitamin and mineral supplements obtained over-the-counter for various reasons: your patients may not think of these supplements as medications and may not mention them when you take a medical history.

Although often perceived as entirely harmless, in some situations use of these supplements may be dangerous. For example, patients on coumarin anti-coagulants like warfarin, should not take vitamin K supplements. Also, pregnant women should avoid taking vitamin A supplements as this may exceed the safe recommended daily dose and cause congenital defects of the foetus.

It is recommended to have a healthy diet and lifestyle to provide the body with micronutrients. However, often diets are suboptimal and may not meet the body's requirements.

In addition to systemic medications and supplements, vitamins and minerals can be added to topical preparations, for example fluoride in toothpastes and oral rinses.

Vitamins occur in two groups: they are classified as either water-soluble or fat-soluble. In humans, there are 13 vitamins: 4 fat-soluble (A, D, E and K) and 9 water-soluble (8 B vitamins and vitamin C). Fat-soluble vitamins are absorbed through the intestinal tract with the help of lipids (fats). Because they are likely to accumulate in the body, they are more likely to lead to hypervitaminosis.

Water-soluble vitamins dissolve readily in water and are easily excreted from the body. Fat and water soluble vitamins will now be discussed in turn. This will be followed by a consideration of minerals and trace elements.

Fat-soluble vitamins

The fat-soluble vitamins will now be discussed in turn. The details relating to individual vitamins are summarized in Table 23.1.

Vitamin A

There are several compounds that have vitamin A activity – retinol, retinoic acid, retinalaldehyde and carotenoids that can be cleaved to yield retinalaldehyde and are sometimes called provitamin A.

Retinol and retinoic acid are found in animal products such as liver, egg yolk, fish liver oil, whole milk. Carotenoids are found in various vegetables and fruit, especially green, yellow and orange vegetables contain beta-carotene.

Retinol and carotene are absorbed from the small intestine and as they are fat-soluble, they require lipids to be absorbed. Low fat diets impair the absorption and can be associated with vitamin A deficiency. On the other hand, most of the dietary retinol gets absorbed and is stored in the liver. Excessive vitamin A intake can lead to hypervitaminosis, which is a serious toxic condition.

Recommended daily allowance (RDA) (or reference nutrient intake, RNI) of vitamin A for adults is 600–700 mcg/day. Vitamin A deficiency in developed countries is rare as liver stores can last 1-3 years. However, in developing countries vitamin A deficiency-related problems are common. Worldwide it is estimated each year about 10 million pre-school children and pregnant women are at risk of developing blindness due to vitamin A deficiency. Initially deficiency impairs vision's adaptation to dim light and night blindness. This is reversible. Prolonged deficiency causes xerophthalmia – severe dryness of eyes leading to ulceration of the cornea and keratinization causing irreversible blindness. Vitamin A is also required for epithelial cell turnover and deficiency produces thickening of skin and mucosae due to hyperkeratosis.

Table 23.1 Summary of fat-soluble vitamins

Vitamin	RNI	Sources	Deficiency	Toxicity	Preparations used in medicine	Importance in dentistry
Vitamin A	600–700 mcg/day	Butter, whole milk, egg yolk, liver, colourful vegetables and fruits	Eyes - Night blindness, xerophthalmia, keratomalacia, irreversible blindness Skin - hyperkeratosis	Hypervitaminosis A - CNS – headache, nausea, ataxia; Liver – hepatomegaly; Bones – joint pain, calcification of soft tissue; Skin – dryness, scaling, hair loss	Isoretinoin, acitretin – dermatology (severe acne, psoriasis)	Topical retinoids occasionally used to treat oral white patches.
Vitamin D	5–15 mcg/day depending on age, latitude and season, skin pigmentation and sun protection	Oily fish, eggs, full fat milk. D₃ is also formed in the skin in sunlight.	Children – rickets (bony deformities – bowed legs, narrow rib cages, short stature. Adults – osteomalacia (demineralization of bones and deformities)	Weakness, nausea, loss of appetite, abdominal pain, diarrhoea, headaches, hypercalcaemia and soft tissue calcification.	Cholecalciferol often in combination with calcium to treat osteporosis.	
Vitamin E	15 mg/day	Oily fish, nuts, seeds, beans, green leafy vegetables	Very rare. Neurological abnormalities. Premature infants - haemolytic anaemia.	Very low toxicity		
Vitamin K	90–120 mcg/day	Liver, leafy green vegetables – broccoli, spinach, kale	Vitmin K deficiency bleeding (VKDB) of infants. Adults – bleeding	No documented. Interferes with anticoagulants	In new-borns to prevent bleeding. To reverse warfarin anticoagulation	

Hypervitaminosis is unlikely to happen due to normal dietary sources, but is possible with supplements and prescribed synthetic retinoids used to treat certain dermatological conditions. An excessive amount of vitamin A is both acutely and chronically toxic. Acute toxicity can cause nausea, vomiting, headache, itching and exfoliation of skin. Prolonged excessive intake can affect the central nervous system, liver, skin and bones. Retinol is teratogenic, hence pregnant women should avoid vitamin A supplements and must not be managed with synthetic retinoids. Carotenoids have limited conversion to retinol and therefore do not cause hypervitaminosis, but can cause cosmetic darkening of skin.

Use in medicine:

Retinoic acid derivates are used topically and systemically in dermatology. Acitretin has a moderating effect on abnormal epithelial differentiation and keratinization. It is used to treat severe forms of psoriasis, congenital ichthyosis and Darier's disease, as well as lichen planus, keratoderma and to prevent malignancy in sun damage. It increases the epithelial turnover. Isotretinoin is used to treat severe acne. It reduces hypercornification, lowers sebum excretion and has an anti-inflammatory effect. Although the exact mechanism is not clear, retinoids have an effect on cell differentiation and inhibit neoplasia and, therefore, are sometimes used to treat dysplastic lesions.

Vitamin D

Vitamin D is a seco-steroid, that can be synthesized in the skin by a cholesterol-like precursor by exposure to sunlight. Due to the fact that it can be made by the body there is debate whether it is a vitamin or a hormone. The version made in the skin is referred to as vitamin D_3 (cholecalciferol). The dietary form can be both D_3 or D_2 (ergocalciferol). From a nutritional perspective both forms are similarly metabolized and equal in potency.

The main physiological role of vitamin D is maintaining calcium balance in the body. It works in conjunction with parathyroid hormone and increases calcium levels in the blood by acting on the intestine, kidney and bone. It also regulates phosphate levels in the blood.

Vitamin D deficiency in children causes rickets, which is characterized by bone weakness and deformities. In adults, vitamin D deficiency presents as osteomalacia, causing bone pain and weakness. Vitamin D overdose can cause nausea, headache, abdominal pain, diarrhoea and hypercalcaemia leading to hypertension and calcification of soft tissues.

Use in medicine:

Vitamin D supplements are used in vitamin D deficiency. Together with calcium supplements they are used to prevent or treat osteoporosis.

Vitamin E

Vitamin E, tocopherol, has an antioxidant function. Although it was thought to slow the ageing processes and reduce the risk of cancer or cardiovascular disease, there is little evidence for this. Vitamin E deficiency is rare. In premature infants it can be associated with haemolytic anaemia. Vitamin E has a very low toxicity.

Use in medicine:

Vitamin E is occasionally used to prevent haemolytic anaemia.

Vitamin K

There are two naturally occurring forms of Vitamin K: phylloquinone from plants (vitamin K_1), and bacterial menaquinone (vitamin K_2) and a synthetic vitamin K_3. Vitamin K is a co-enzyme needed for synthesis of clotting factors such as prothrombin. It is also needed in production of proteins involved in bone re-modelling.

Use in medicine:

Newborns are given an intramuscular vitamin K injection to prevent bleeding. It can be used to reverse the anticoagulant effect of warfarin.

Water-soluble vitamins

The water-soluble vitamins are comprised of the B vitamins and vitamin C. The details relating to individual vitamins are summarized in Table 23.2.

Table 23.2 Summary of water-soluble vitamins

Vitamin	RNI	Sources	Deficiency	Use in medicine	Use in dentistry
Vitamin B$_1$ (Thiamine)	1.1–1.2 mg/day	Grains, seeds, nuts, pork	Beriberi, Wernicke's encephalopathy	In alcohol abuse to prevent encephalopathy or Korsakoff syndrome	
Vitamin B$_2$ (Riboflavin)	1.1–1.3 mg/day	Milk, liver, red meat, poultry, grains, asparagus, broccoli, spinach	Angular cheilitis, glossitis, skin rash		
Vitamin B$_3$ (Nicoti-namide, nicotinic acid, niacin)	1.5 mg/day	Beef, chicken, fish, whole grains	Pellegra	In dermatology in management of acne, immunobullous diseases	In Oral Medicine in management of vesiculobullous disorders
Vitamin B$_6$ (Pyridoxine)	1.3 mg/day	Chicken, fish, pork, brown rice, seeds, broccoli, spinach, banana	Headaches, confusion, seizures, poor growth	Premenstrual syndrome, carpal tunnel syndrome	
Vitamin B$_{12}$ (Cobalamin)	1.5mcg/day	Meat, fish, milk	Pernicious anaemia, macrocytic anaemia, oral ulcers, neuropathy		In Oral Medicine if underlying deficiency causing oral ulceration, glossitis and burning sensation
Folate (Folic acid; vitamin B$_9$)	200 mcg/day (400 mcg/day in pregnancy)	Leafy green vegetables, seeds, lentils, liver	Macrocytic anaemia, glossitis, oral ulcers, neural tube defects	In pregnancy to prevent neural tube defects	In Oral Medicine if underlying deficiency causing oral ulceration, glossitis and burning sensation
Vitamin C (ascorbic acid)	25–40 mg/day	Citrus fruit, strawberries, peppers, leafy green vegetables	Scurvy		

Vitamin B$_5$, Pantothenic acid, and vitamin B$_7$, Biotin, have no routine therapeutic uses and are not discussed further

Vitamin B$_1$

Vitamin B$_1$ or thiamine was the first vitamin to be identified. It is widely distributed in foods. It is important in energy metabolism and in metabolism of amino acids. Deficiency develops rapidly and can result in chronic peripheral neuritis (dry beriberi), acute pernicious beriberi with heart failure and Wernicke's encephalopathy, associated with alcohol abuse. No toxicity of high doses of vitamin B$_1$ has been reported.

Vitamin B$_2$

Vitamin B$_2$ or riboflavin is essential in energy metabolism and is also involved in converting various other vitamins in their active forms. Riboflavin is important for tissue repair and wound healing. Deficiency can cause angular cheilitis and glossitis, however it is rarely seen in isolation and is seen in conjunction with other vitamin deficiencies.

Vitamin B$_3$

Niacin is the generic term of the two vitamin compounds, nicotinic acid and nicotinamide. It is involved in energy metabolism. It also has anti-inflammatory properties such as neutrophil and eosinophil chemotaxis, secretion of inflammatory mediators and inhibition of IgE-related histamine release.

Deficiency causes pellagra, which is characterized by photosensitive dermatitis, diarrhoea, memory problems and psychosis. Untreated pellagra can be fatal. Excessive doses of niacin can cause flushing, nausea and itching.

Use in medicine:

Nicotinamide is used in dermatology for its anti-inflammatory effect in management of acne vulgaris, acne rosacea and vesicullobullous conditions such as pemphigoid.

Vitamin B$_6$

Vitamin B$_6$ includes 6 vitamers that are metabolically interconvertible and have equal biological activities. It has multiple roles in amino acid metabolism, lipid metabolism and in steroid hormone actions. Vitamin B$_6$ is available in various foods and also synthesized by intestinal flora, therefore severe deficiency is rare. No adverse effects are known from high vitamin B$_6$ intake from food, however excessive amounts of supplements can cause peripheral sensory neuropathy.

Use in medicine:

It has been suggested vitamin B$_6$ has a role in reducing cardiovascular risk, possibly by reducing elevated homocysteine levels. Although there is little evidence, vitamin B$_6$ supplements are used in premenstrual syndrome, carpal tunnel syndrome and boosting immunity.

Folate

The term folate includes a number of compounds. Folic acid strictly refers only to one form. All forms of folate can be found in food, however folic acid is typically used to fortify food and can be taken as a supplement. Folate has an important role in DNA synthesis, and is particularly important for rapidly dividing cells in bone marrow producing red blood cells, mucosa, skin, and in development of the embryo.

Folate deficiency can cause anaemia and poor growth. In the oral cavity, it can cause ulceration, glossitis and a burning sensation. Folate deficiency in early pregnancy increases the risk of neural tube defects of the embryo. Certain groups are at risk of folate deficiency: pregnant women, premature infants, malnourished people, alcoholics and tobacco smokers. High doses of folate supplements can mask co-existing B$_{12}$ deficiency and increases risk of undetected B$_{12}$ deficiency leading to irreversible neurological damage.

Use in medicine:

Folic acid supplements are advised for women trying to conceive and during pregnancy. Some medications, such as methotrexate, cause folate deficiency and therefore require supplementation between doses to protect the patient from, for example oral ulceration.

Vitamin B$_{12}$

Vitamin B$_{12}$ has various vitamers. It plays a role in the metabolism of methionine, fatty acids and leucine. It is found almost exclusively in animal products. It can be synthesized by fungi, bacteria and algae, and accumulates in animal tissue. Human colon microflora produce B$_{12}$, but it is not absorbed. Vitamin B$_{12}$ has to be first released from food by acids in the stomach. In the small intestine it binds to intrinsic factors produced by parietal cells in the stomach and gets absorbed. Only a small amount can be absorbed without intrinsic factor. B$_{12}$ is secreted by bile, but most of it is reabsorbed. Due to this efficient store and reuse, deficiency due to poor intake can take a few years to manifest. Severe B$_{12}$ deficiency due to malabsorption can occur in autoimmune destruction of gastric parietal cells that produce intrinsic factor.

Deficiency can cause secondary folate deficiency resulting in macrocytic anaemia. It also infers with the maintenance of myelin in nerve coatings resulting in multiple neurological disorders. If untreated, severe vitamin B_{12} deficiency can be fatal, hence the name 'pernicious anaemia'.

Use in medicine:

Vitamin B_{12} oral supplements and intramuscular injections are used in B_{12} deficiency. If the deficiency is due to autoimmune disorder, the therapy is life-long.

Vitamin C

Vitamin C or ascorbic acid is present in various fruits (e.g. citrus fruit, kiwi fruit, melon, apple), berries (e.g. strawberries, blackcurrants), and vegetables (e.g. broccoli, peppers, cabbage, tomatoes, potatoes). However, it is unstable and can be destroyed by heat, light and oxygen. It is important for the synthesis of collagen and catecholamines. Vitamin C is an antioxidant and can protect cells from damage caused by free radicals. It also increases iron absorption from food through reduction from the ferric to ferrous form.

Vitamin C deficiency can lead to scurvy, historically seen in sailors and armies due to lack of fresh fruit and vegetables. It presents as poor wound healing, pin-point bleeding, joint aches, fractures, fatigue and mood changes. Intra-orally it can cause gingivitis, gum bleeding and loose teeth. Often there is co-existent iron deficiency anaemia due to poor absorption. Nowadays scurvy is rare in developed countries, however vitamin C deficiency can be observed in individuals with poor diet.

Although vitamin C is considered non-toxic, excessive doses can cause gastric irritation. Also, excessive amounts increase iron absorption and can interact with anticoagulants. Chewable vitamin C supplements can cause enamel acid erosion.

Minerals and trace elements

Minerals are inorganic elements essential to structural and physiological functions of the body. If a mineral dietary intake needs to be greater than 100 mg/day, it is considered to be a major mineral, for example calcium, phosphorus and magnesium. If the dietary intake required is less than 100 mg/day, it is considered to be a trace element, for example iron, zinc, iodine and selenium. Both major minerals and trace elements are important for maintaining a healthy body and deficiencies can be equally damaging.

Calcium and phosphorus

Calcium is the most abundant mineral in the body providing the structure of the bones and teeth. Both calcium and phosphorus form hydroxyapatite, the major inorganic bone component. They also have a role in cell signalling, coagulation and energy metabolism. Calcium metabolism is controlled by parathyroid hormone, calcitriol and calcitonin. Calcium deficiency can lead to osteoporosis. In children with developing teeth, low calcium levels can cause enamel defects. In Western diet the main source of calcium is dairy products. Smaller amounts of calcium can be found in green vegetables and grains.

Use in medicine:

Calcium supplements are used to prevent or treat osteoporosis. Often these are combined with vitamin D.

Iron

Iron is an essential trace element with numerous biochemical roles. Iron is essential for haemoglobin that carries oxygen from the lungs to the tissues. In the diet, it comes from both animal and plant sources. Meat, poultry and fish are good sources of haeme iron. Leafy green vegetables and grains contain non-haeme iron. Iron deficiency can lead to microcytic anaemia, which can have oral manifestations such as mouth ulcers, angular cheilitis, a burning sensation and glossitis.

Use in medicine:

Iron supplements are used to treat or prevent iron deficiency.

Fluoride

The main role of fluoride is mineralization of bones and teeth by forming calcium fluoroapatite. At varying levels fluoride is present in most foods and water. In the areas with low fluoride content in the water it can be added to the drinking water to prevent dental caries. Fluoride is toxic. Small amounts of excessive intake can lead to fluorosis of developing teeth and the skeleton. High excessive doses of fluoride can cause renal damage, gastrointestinal, neurological and cardiovascular disturbance and can even be lethal.

Use in public health:

Fluoride can be added to the drinking water.

Use in dentistry:

Fluoride is added to tooth pastes and mouth rinses to prevent dental caries by making enamel more resistant to acid and helping to remineralize softened enamel. Fluoride-containing gels and varnishes containing high doses of fluoride are used by dental health professionals to prevent caries.

CHAPTER 24

Musculoskeletal therapeutics

Martyn Ormond

Key Topics

- Overview of musculoskeletal disorders
- Common drugs used in the management of musculoskeletal disorders and their pharmacology
- Implications for dentistry

Learning Objectives

- To describe the pharmacological management of musculoskeletal disorders
- To understand the main drug categories and describe their mechanism of action, indications and adverse effects
- To understand the implications of dentistry

Essential Dental Therapeutics, First Edition. Edited by David Wray.
© 2018 John Wiley & Sons Ltd. Published 2018 by John Wiley & Sons Ltd.
Companion Website: www.wiley.com/go/wray/dental-therapeutics

Introduction

Musculoskeletal disorders include a wide range of diseases such as osteoarthritis and rheumatoid arthritis as well as the spondyloarthropathies and gout. Although the aetiology and presentations vary, they all result in inflammation that leads to tissue damage.

Acute inflammation describes the rapid response of the innate immune system to a challenge. It comprises of a cellular component (leucocytes, macrophages, mast cells, natural killer cells and endothelial cells), plasma proteins (including the complement, coagulation, fibrinolytic and kinin systems) and mediators (such as histamine, eicosanoids, cytokines, chemokines and nitric oxide).

Inflammation becomes chronic when the initiating trigger is not eradicated or the individual exhibits a susceptibility to prolonging the inflammatory process. Chronic inflammatory conditions such as rheumatoid arthritis involve interaction between the innate and adaptive immune response. The adaptive immune response involves both T and B lymphocytes. It is highly specific, resulting in the production of antibodies to an antigen. In chronic inflammatory diseases this process may become self-perpetuating.

This chapter will consider the aetiopathogenesis of these musculoskeletal disorders followed by a consideration of the relevant therapeutic agents used to treat them.

Musculoskeletal disorders

The most common of these disorders are: osteoarthritis, rheumatoid arthritis, the spondyloarthropathies and gout. These will be discussed in turn.

Osteoarthritis

Osteoarthritis (OA) is the most common disease of synovial joints leading to pain and disability. It is the result of aging and trauma on bone and cartilage within the joint. By the age of 60 years approximately half of the population will be affected by OA, with weight bearing joints such as the hips and knees most commonly involved. Treatment is directed towards pain management and preventing disease progression. This involves a combination of drugs, physical interventions (e.g. weight loss), exercises, aids (e.g. walking sticks) and surgery if necessary. Simple analgesics such as paracetamol are the first-line therapy followed by non-steroidal anti-inflammatory drugs (NSAIDs). However intra-articular corticosteroids many be required for inflammatory exacerbations.

Rheumatoid arthritis

Rheumatoid arthritis (RA) affects 2–3% of the population with three times as many women affected as men. It is a systemic disease characterized by a symmetrical inflammatory deforming polyarthropathy in addition to many extra-articular manifestations. The peak age of onset is between 30 and 40 years. However, it can present at any age. The aetiology is most likely autoimmune. There is often a strong family history and an association with HLA-DR4.

It often initially affects the small joints of the hands and feet before progressing to involve larger joints. The joints become stiff and swollen, eventually this may lead to subluxation and deformities. This is the result of erosion of bone, cartilage and tendons by an inflammatory pannus comprising of T lymphocytes and polymorphonuclear leucocytes leading to chronic synovitis.

RA management includes exercise and physiotherapy to maintain function and prevent deformities. Surgery may be required to correct deformities. Drug treatment aims to control symptoms and modify the underlying inflammatory process. Simple analgesics and NSAIDs are widely used in addition to disease-modifying anti-rheumatoid drugs (DMARDs) such as sulfasalazine, methotrexate and azathioprine. Patients with moderate to severe disease now often progress to the use of cytokine inhibitors such as infliximab and adalimumab or TNF α blockers such as etanercept.

The spondarthropathies

Spondyloarthropathies include a number of diseases such as ankylosing spondylitis, reactive arthritis, enteropathic arthropathies, psoriatic arthritis and juvenile chronic arthritis. There is often a strong family history as well as an association with HLA-B27.

Ankylosing spondylitis:

This typically affects young men. It presents with sacroiliitis causing pain in the buttocks which radiates down the back of the legs. This leads to spinal fusion with limitation of movement, low back pain and morning stiffness.

Psoriatic arthritis:

This occurs in 10% of patients with psoriasis affecting the small joints of the hands asymmetrically. Treatment includes analgesics and often immunosuppressant drugs.

Enteropathic arthropathy:

This occurs in patients with inflammatory bowel disease. It typically affects the knees and ankles as a monoarthritis or asymmetrical oligoarthritis. Management involves treating the underlying inflammatory bowel disease.

Gout

Gout is a crystal arthropathy arising from the deposition of sodium urate crystals in joints and soft tissue due to an abnormality of uric acid metabolism. There is either an overproduction or underexcretion of uric acid resulting in hyperuricaemia. There are many causes including idiopathic, drugs, renal impairment, hypertension and alcohol.

Acute attacks usually present as a red, hot, swollen and painful first toe although it can also affect the ankle, wrist or knee. This can lead to joint erosions and deformity and chronic tophaceous gout in which there is deposition of urate in the soft tissues and around joints.

During an acute attack, high dose NSAIDs, or alternatively colchicine, are given. Recurrent or chronic gout can be treated prophylactically with allopurinol. This can trigger an acute attack and therefore NSAIDs or colchicine is given for the first month of treatment.

Drugs used for musculoskeletal disorders

There is a range of therapeutic agents that is effective in the management of musculoskeletal disorders as detailed below.

Non-steroidal anti-inflammatory drugs (NSAIDs)

NSAIDs are widely used analgesics that also exert anti-inflammatory actions. They are a chemically heterogeneous group of chemicals that work by inhibiting cyclo-oxygenase (COX). COX catalyses the synthesis of prostaglandins and thromboxane from arachidonic acid. Most cells express the isoform COX-1 whereas COX-2 is induced when activated by inflammatory cells. The inhibition of COX-1 affects the production of prostaglandins required for normal tissue homeostasis resulting in a number of adverse effects. NSAIDs are classified as COX-2 selective (coxib drugs) which selectively inhibit COX-2 or COX-1 and non COX-2 selective compounds (all other drugs).

The three main therapeutic actions of NSAIDs are: analgesic, antipyretic and anti-inflammatory. Each drug varies in the degree to which it demonstrates each action, for example while ibuprofen exhibits all three actions, paracetamol does not possess anti-inflammatory properties.

Aspirin:

Aspirin (acetylsalicylic acid) is rarely used in musculoskeletal disorders due to its side-effect profile. Its anti-inflammatory effects are mediated through its inhibition of COX-2. However due to its effect on prostaglandin production, essential for gastric protection, it is not used in the context of musculoskeletal conditions. Additionally it is known to cause hypersensitivity reactions.

Paracetamol:

Paracetamol (acetaminophen) is extensively used in musculoskeletal conditions for its analgesic properties. It is absorbed via the small intestine with a half-life of 2 hours. It is metabolized in the liver and excreted via the kidneys. It has little anti-inflammatory actions. The side-effect profile is relatively unremarkable with the exception of the consequences of a paracetamol overdose which may be only twice the recommended therapeutic dose. This can lead to significant hepatoxicity and major organ failure ultimately leading to death.

Propionic acid derivatives:

These drugs include ibuprofen and naproxen. They are rapidly absorbed and have a half-life of 2 hours. They are almost entirely bound to proteins, metabolized in the liver and excreted through the kidneys. They have a similar side-effect profile as aspirin, including hypersensitivity reactions, however they are generally well tolerated and used extensively in musculoskeletal disorders. They should be avoided in those with asthma as they may exacerbate bronchospasm.

Corticosteroids

Corticosteroids, specifically glucocortoids, are potent anti-inflammatory drugs that are used routinely in a wide range of chronic inflammatory conditions, including rheumatoid arthritis. Their effect is due to their ability to alter the activity of corticosteroid-responsive genes. This results in a decrease in arachidoinc acid formation by inducing lipocortin which inhibits phospholipase A_2. This prevents the production of all downstream pro-inflammatory products including leukotrienes and prostaglandins. Additionally glucorticoids reduce the number and also activity of immune cells, such as lymphocytes, neutrophils and macrophages. This effect on macrophages as well as fibroblasts is particularly important in chronic inflammation.

There are many adverse effects associated with the prolonged use of glucorticoids. As a result they are mainly used in the initial management of an inflammatory condition to induce disease control or in the management of acute flares. The osteoporotic effects of corticosteroids also limit their usefulness in arthritic disorders.

Colchicine

Colchicine is used primarily for acute attacks of gout. It inhibits microtubule assembly by binding to tubulin (the protein monomer of microtubules).

This prevents cytoskeletal movements and cell motility preventing leucocyte migration. It additionally decreases the release of histamine by mast cells through the same mechanism.

It is given orally and is rapidly effective. Its main side effects relate to gastrointestinal toxicity, with nausea, vomiting and diarrhoea. Rarely, chronic use of colchicine can lead to agranulocytosis and aplastic anaemia.

Allopurinol

Prophylactic prevention of acute gout attacks involves drugs that reduce uric acid production such as allopurinol. Allopurinol inhibits the enzyme xanthine oxidase which converts xanthine and hypoxanthine (products of DNA breakdown) to uric acid. It is absorbed by the gut, metabolized by the liver and excreted by the kidney.

Adverse effects such as headaches, diarrhoea, rash and acute exacerbation of gout have been reported. Rarely it may cause acute allergic reactions. It is associated with a number of drug interactions, most notably with azathioprine.

Disease-modifying anti-rheumatic drugs (DMARDs)

These drugs comprise a diverse group of agents effective in the management of rheumatoid arthritis and other musculoskeletal disorders. They will now be considered in turn.

Sulfasalazine:

Sulfasalazine is broken down in the gut by commensal colonic bacteria to sulfapyridine and 5-aminosalicylate acid (5-ASA). Sulfapyridine decreases synovial IL-8 production and inhibits angiogenesis thought to be important in the management of rheumatoid arthritis. However 5-ASA is thought to be mainly responsible for its anti-inflammatory properties as it inhibits cyclooxygenase and lipo-oxygenase, scavenges free radicals and inhibits the production of pro-inflammatory cytokines and immunoglobulins.

Adverse reactions include nausea, vomiting, headaches and rashes. It may lead to blood disorders and, rarely, cause allergic reactions.

Methotrexate:

Methotrexate is a folic acid antagonist. It disrupts dihydrofolate reductase which is required for purine synthesis and therefore DNA synthesis. It is widely used in rheumatoid arthritis and psoriatic arthritis as well as a number of other chronic inflammatory diseases.

It is given orally once weekly with folic acid given either three times weekly or on all days except when methotrexate is given in order to minimize its side effect profile.

Methotrexate may cause bone marrow toxicity as well as hepatotoxicity and pulmonitis. Additionally, it is associated with mouth ulcers and gastrointestinal disturbances which are minimized by the addition of folic acid. It should not be taken during pregnancy, as it is embryotoxic.

Azathioprine:

Azathioprine is a prodrug that is converted to 6-mercaptopurine in the liver. It triggers apoptosis and inhibits purine synthesis particularly in proliferating lymphocytes. Before prescribing it is necessary to assess the levels of the liver enzyme thiopurine methyltransferase (TPMT), as it is important in the drug's metabolism and levels may vary between individual patients.

Azathioprine has a number of adverse effects such as bone marrow suppression with leucopenia and thrombocytopenia, increased susceptibility to infection, hepatotoxicity, nausea, alopecia and an increased risk of malignancy.

There are a number of important drug interactions. Both sulfasalazine and NSAIDs inhibit TPMT and therefore azathioprine metabolism. Allopurinol inhibits xanthine oxidase, which again leads to decreased drug metabolism increasing the risk of toxicity. When used with angiotensin-converting enzyme inhibitors there is an increased risk of myelosuppression.

Mycophenolate mofetil:

Mycophenolate mofetil is metabolized to mycophenolic acid, which inhibits monophosphate dehydrogenase, essential for lymphocyte proliferation. It is prescribed off licence as a second-line agent in the treatment of a number of chronic inflammatory conditions. It can lead to bone marrow suppression and increases the risk of infection and, potentially, malignancies. More commonly, patients report gastrointestinal disturbances similar to azathioprine.

Hydroxychloroquine:

Hydroxychloroquine is widely used in systemic lupus erythematosis and other connective tissue diseases however it is often used as an adjunct in rheumatoid arthritis. Its exact mechanism of action is unknown although it can reduce the production of pro-inflammatory cytokines, including TNFα, interferon and IL-6. In addition, it inhibits the acidification of lysosomes that may decrease T cell activation by altering antigen procession and presentation.

The side effect profile includes nausea and gastrointestinal disturbance, headache, rash, alopecia and, rarely, it may cause blood dyscrasias. It should be avoided in patients with hepatic and renal impairment as well as those with glucose-6-phosphate dehydrogenase deficiency. Rarely it is associated with retinal toxicity and yearly visual testing is recommenced.

Gold:

The use of gold in rheumatoid arthritis has decreased significantly since the introduction of methotrexate and the anti-TNFα agents. It can be given either orally or by intramuscular injection and is thought to affect chemotaxis and phagocytosis of macrophages.

Adverse effects include mouth ulcers, lichenoid reactions, rash, skin pigmentation, proteinuria, blood dyscrasias, hepatitis, peripheral neuropathy and pulmonary infiltrates. It should be avoided in those with hepatitis or renal disease as well as during pregnancy and when breastfeeding.

Biological agents – anti-TNFα agents

TNFα is an important pro-inflammatory cytokine produced mainly by macrophages although T helper CD4+ cells also contribute. It activates macrophages to eradicate intracellular bacterial and fungal infections. TNFα also contributes to the pathogenesis of a number of chronic inflammatory conditions such as rheumatoid arthritis and Crohn's disease.

Infliximab is a humanized monoclonal IgG1 antibody given by infusion whereas adalimumab is a fully human monoclonal IgG1 antibody which is given by subcutaneous injection. Etanercept differs slightly in that it is a recombinant molecule consisting of 2 human p75 TNFα receptors attached to the Fc component of human IgG1. It is also given by subcutaneous injection.

Each of the anti-TNFα drugs results in an increased susceptibility to infections by intracellular microorganisms, particularly tuberculosis. Infliximab may be associated with infusion reactions since it is chimeric, with patients experiencing fevers, pruritis, urticarial, hypotension and dyspnoea. All anti-TNFα drugs in theory increase the risk of malignancy, particularly lymphomas.

Dental relevance

Analgesics are widely used in musculoskeletal disorders as well as for the management of dental pain and so patients may be at risk of taking these drugs simultaneously for concurrent conditions. While the majority are safe with few significant side effects there are a number of important considerations.

Paracetamol is a useful analgesic in dentistry and is a safe drug when used correctly. However this may lead to the misconception that it can be used without concern. When only twice the maximum therapeutic dose is taken it results in paracetamol toxicity. This can cause irreparable liver damage and ultimately prove fatal. Overdose is a medical emergency and should de dealt with swiftly; ideally

treatment should be commenced within 12 hours of the excessive dose.

NSAIDs have numerous unwanted adverse effects however there are few important to dentistry. The exception is aspirin due to its irreversible inhibition of platelet cyclo-oxygenase leading to the risk of post-operative bleeding.

Both NSAIDs and a number of DMARDs, including hydroxychloroquine, gold salts and sulfasalazine may cause oral lichenoid reactions. These are clinically indistinguishable from idiopathic lichen planus. In some patients this may require giving consideration to changing the causative DMARD although in some patients it may be necessary to continue the drug and the oral complications must be managed. DMARDs such as methotrexate may cause oral ulcers and gold salts have been reported as causing taste disturbances.

Drugs used in chronic inflammatory musculoskeletal disorders often involve suppression of the immune system, including corticosteroids, many of the DMARDs and all of the anti-TNFα agents. It the dental setting this most commonly results in an increase in oral infections, particularly viral and fungal infections. Oral candidosis can prove challenging to treat with limited response to therapy and relapse. Viral infections, typically herpes group viruses (HSV and CMV) can be seen and may require both active and prophylactic treatment. Immunosuppression increases the risk of malignancy, although the effect of immunosuppressant drugs is unclear. The most common malignancies associated with immunosuppression include lymphomas and squamous cell carcinomas. Dentists should be vigilant for any evidence of a developing malignancy and refer as appropriate.

Index

repaglinide, 123
reproductive hormones, 115–116
respiratory disease, 138–141
respiratory disease medications,
    141–143
    implications for dentistry,
        143–144
    long-acting agents, 141
    short-acting agents, 141
respiratory physiology, 138
respiratory syncytial virus (RSV)
        infections, 51–52
rheumatoid arthritis, 176
rhinitis, 139, 141, 142
ribavirin, 51–52
rifampicin, 34, 36, 40
rilpivirine, 50
riluzole, 98
ringworm (tinea), 44
risperidone, 90, 92, 105
Ritalin, 106
ritonavir, 50–51
rivaroxaban, 152
rivastigmine, 96
root canal treatment, antiseptics,
    24, 25
ropivacaine, 59
rosuvastatin, 132
rotavirus, 27
routes of drug administration, 12

S
salbutamol, 4, 17, 78, 79–80, 141
saliva, 74
salmeterol, 141
salt, fluoridated, 70
saquinavir, 50–51
SBAR (Situation, Background,
        Assessment,
        Recommendation)
        approach, 78
schizophrenia, 104–105
    antipsychotic drugs, 105
    considerations within the dental
        clinic, 105
    drug interactions with dental
        medications, 105
    environmental risk factors,
        104–105
    functional changes in the brain,
        105
    genetic component, 104

role of dopamine, 105
side effects of medications, 105
scurvy, 173
sedative medications, 92
seizures, 82, 102–104
selective serotonin reuptake
        inhibitors (SSRIs), 5, 88, 92
selective toxicity, 5–6
serotonin and noradrenaline
        reuptake inhibitors
        (SNRIs), 62, 88, 92
sevoflurane, 58–59
shingles, 49
simvastatin, 132
sinusitis, antibiotics, 33
Sjögren's syndrome, 76
skin, fungal infections, 44
social anxiety disorder (SAD), 91
sodium hypochlorite (bleach), 25,
        29
sofosbuvir, 48
sotalol, 131
spironolactone, 132
spondylarthropathies, 176–177
St John's wort (*Hypericum
        perforatum*), 18, 88
Staphylococcus spp. infections, 32
statins, 132
status epilepticus, 82
stavudine, 50
stem cell transplants, 164
sterilization, definition, 24
steroids *see* corticosteroids
steroid-sparing agents, for
        inflammatory bowel disease,
        157
Stevens-Johnson syndrome, 38
stimulants (for constipation), 156
streptomycin, 34, 40
stroke, 94–95, 128
    impact on oral hygiene and oral
        health, 95–96
sucralfate, 155
sulfasalazine, 158, 178
sulfonamide drugs, 5, 17, 21, 34, 36
sulfonamide-trimethoprim
        combinations,
        pharmacokinetics, 37–38
sulfonylureas, 123
sunitinib, 162
surface cleaning agents, 27
suxamethonium, 20, 58

syncope, 83–84
systemic corticosteroids, 67–68
    equivalent dosages, 67
    prednisolone, 67
    procedures requiring steroid
        cover, 68
    prophylactic treatments, 67
    side effects, 67

T
tea tree oil (*Melaleuca alternifolia*),
        29
teicoplanin, 39
telaprevir, 48
telbivuidine, 48
telmisartan, 129
temazepam, 60, 92
temporomandibular disorder
        (TMD), pain related to, 55
tenofovir disoproxil, 48, 50
teratogens, 18
terbinafine, 45–46
tetrabenazine, 98
tetracyclines, 5, 12, 34, 35–36, 38
thalidomide, 16, 163
theophylline, 142
theophylline ethylenediamine, 142
therapeutic index for drugs, 16
therapeutic range of drugs, 8
therapeutics
    current challenges, 2
    empirico-rational approach, 2–3
    historical basis in natural potions,
        2, 3
    history of development, 2–3
    magico-religious approach, 2, 3
    role in dentistry, 2
thiazide diuretics, 132
thiazolidinediones, 123
thrombocythaemia, 148
thrombocytopenia, 148
thrombocytosis, 148
thrush (pseudomembranous
        candidiasis), 43–44
thymol, 25, 29
thyroid gland disorders, 111–112
thyroid storm, 112
thyrotoxicosis, 111–112
ticarcillin, 34
tinea (ringworm), 44
tioconazole, 45
tiotropium, 141–142